WHY I T ABOUT URINE

... AND A TREATMENT FOR POLYCYSTIC KIDNEY DISEASE

BY JARED JAMES GRANTHAM, MD

BOOKS BY THE AUTHOR

Ashley and the Mooncorn People

Ashley and the Dollmaker

Physiology of the Kidney

Problems in the Diagnosis and Treatment of Polycystic Kidney Disease

The characters and events in this book are real. The author strove to record an accurate accounting of his life with careful attention to time, place and person. If the author has incorrectly described any events or incorrectly imputed the words or deeds of others, living or dead, it was without intent or malice.

Cover and interior art by Roura Young, Lawrence, Kan.

Copyediting by Diane McLendon, Portland, Ore.

Design by Sarah Mosher, Shawnee, Kan.

Published by Rockhill Books,
an imprint of Kansas City Star Books, Kansas City, Mo.

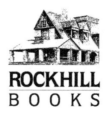

ROCKHILL
B O O K S

For Carol Elaine and Janeane Marie, Jared Taylor, James Aaron and Joel Don and our grandchildren, Ashley Laine, Joshua Lance, Lindsay Taylor, Connor Joel, Addison Marie, Emily Kathleen, Allissa Joel, Elaina Marie, Dillon James, Aidan Michael and great-grandson, Michael Gage.

IN CELEBRATION OF URINE

Who in their right mind would spend any time thinking about urine? Just ask physicians (nephrologists, urologists) and laboratory-based scientists who remain fascinated for life by the wonderfully complex and hidden processes in kidneys that quietly convert blood into urine, keeping us alive and well through this effort.

In "Why I Think About Urine," Jared James Grantham takes you on his life journey shaped by unexpected, and often unwanted, events that led to the discovery of the first effective treatment for a lethal, inherited kidney disease.

A close friend in elementary school privately discloses that he has polycystic disease (PKD) that will one day take his life, a message that will spring into the author's consciousness years later in his kidney research laboratory within hours after he has made a surprising and controversial discovery.

The powerful narrative relating how the twists, turns, bits and pieces of the scientific quest fall in line over many decades to compose a new, international movement to conquer a dreadful kidney disease strains the boundaries of serendipity.

ABOUT THE AUTHOR

Jared James Grantham, M.D. was born in Dodge City, Kansas, and educated in Stanton County Community High School, Baker University and The University of Kansas Medical Center. An internationally recognized, award-winning physician scientist, he is University Distinguished Professor (emeritus) and Founding Director (emeritus) of The Kidney Institute at the University of Kansas Medical Center.

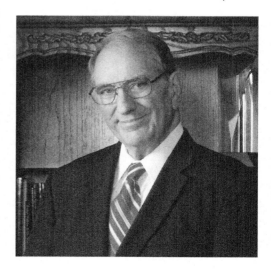

Dr. Grantham has written or co-authored four books on renal disease and two children's books: "Ashley and the Mooncorn People" and "Ashley and the Dollmaker."

ACKNOWLEDGEMENTS

I am indebted to my parents, Jimmie and Ista Grantham, who committed their lives to caring for their children and grandchildren during years of great sacrifice.

I am indebted to the citizens of Johnson City, Kansas, for kind support during some very dark days of my youth.

I am indebted to my sister, Annetta, for brightening my spirit when I lived in Johnson City and for her enduring love.

I thank the Kansas University Medical Center for providing a place to chase my dreams for 55 years, and especially to my academic father, Paul R. Schloerb, MD, a quintessential gentleman and scholar.

I prayerfully remember my deceased childhood friends, Ronnie Wilkerson and Donnie Richard, for precious memories of youth that drove me forward on days when it seemed that the sun would not dare to rise.

I am indebted to Larry Matthews, Dr. Roslyn Coleman, Connie Fowler, Dr. Curt Fowler and Dr. James P. Calvet for reading the manuscript and offering suggestions for improvement, and to Diane Linshaw for finding a frightful number of punctuation and grammatical glitches that would have turned Elsie Hively's hair green.

Finally, I want to praise the memory of my friend and colleague Joseph H. Bruening for creating the Polycystic Kidney Disease Foundation and opening it to the millions of patients around the world who, through the urgency of their needs, continue to inspire physicians and scientists to do all that we can to relieve their suffering.

PREFACE

In your lifetime, you will interrupt what you are doing about 150,000 times to sit on or stand at a toilet and discharge 10,000 gallons of urine, give or take a few drops.

If you are typical, this perfunctory act will consume about 7,000 hours (10 months) of your life as you stare blankly at a wall in a small room or stall. You could have been thinking about urine.

Most of us pay little attention to the organs that make urine. Buried high on the backside of the abdomen on either side of the spine just beneath the rib cage, our kidneys are unbelievably complex, mysterious and, arguably, romantic machines that whiz away day after day unknown and unappreciated. By contrast, the heart, a relatively simple four-chamber pump that could have been designed by an elementary school biology student, makes sounds heard by lovers when an ear is firmly pressed against the chest. For some (Valentine's Day devotees come to mind), the heart is still the seat of the soul. The abandoned kidneys are infinitely more exotic and were they to audibly gurgle or slosh as urine rushes through narrow passageways on its way to the urinary bladder, history might have adopted a different organ symbolizing affection. "I love you with all of my kidney!" Or, "Deep in my kidney." To nephrologists, including me, these are more meaningful terms of endearment.

I am a physician trained in Internal Medicine and Nephrology. Most people I am introduced to have heard of the Internal Medicine part — my mother called them "diagnosticians." Nephrology is what usually stumps them.

"I'm sorry, but I don't know what that is?" is a typical query I hear in impromptu conversations while standing in receiving lines or airport security queues. My short response is, "Nephrologists are internists who spend most of their adult lives thinking about urine." Invariably, my new acquaintance grimaces or turns up his/her nose, giving me *entre*

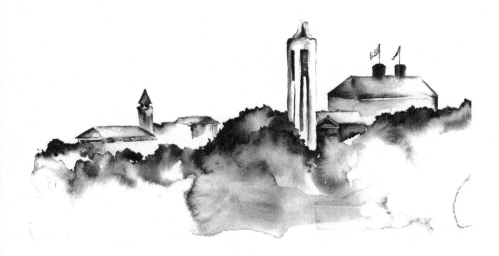

to educate another of the billions of people who have no idea what nephrologists do for a living.

"Is that urology?" is a common follow up question by the quarry.

"No," I reply. "Urologists are surgeons who biopsy prostates. Nephrologists are internists. We biopsy kidneys. So it's fair to say that nephrologists are a 'cut above' urologists."

A disclaimer for potential readers. If, as dowager Countess Grantham of "Downton Abbey," you winced when Dr. Clarkson mentioned urine before a gathering of family members worried about Sybil's toxemia, then I advise you to put this book aside. For you will find that it is a very "nasty" testament to a wondrous, biologic fluid. My hope is that after reading this book, you will become an advocate for the kidneys, urine and the nephrologists who serve this branch of medicine. If this memoir succeeds, kidneys and Nephrology will escape from the "Rodney Dangerfield list of *Organs and Professions of No Respect*" and elevate to a height of veneration.

Jared James Grantham, MD, FACP
Leawood, Kansas

CONTENTS

"Superficially, it might be said that the function of the kidneys is to make urine; but in a more considered view one can say that the kidneys make the stuff of philosophy itself."

— *Homer W. Smith, ScD (1953),*
the father of modern Nephrology

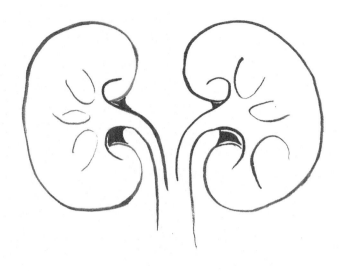

CHAPTER 1

Making first urine

My romance with kidneys began in Dodge City on the dry, wind-blown and dusty plains of western Kansas, when one of my father's intrepid sperm beat out several million of its sibling competitors and burrowed its way into my mother's awaiting egg. That fertilized egg divided into two, four, eight and on up to millions of cells that eventually formed my embryo. Within 12 weeks, my newly minted kidneys had started to function and were forcing the first few drops of urine into my tiny bladder to be quickly squirted into the amniotic cavity, the sac of fluid in which I floated languidly for several months.

For reasons that are not entirely clear, ancient physicians and sooth-sayers referred to the kidney work product as "urine" and the act of passing it outside the body "urination." It also became known as "piss" and the physical act "pissing." The educated gentry have stuck with the more mellow terms "urine" and "urination," whereas in pubs and brothels you are more likely to hear "piss and pissing" or "pee and peeing." Nephrologists, kidney specialists who are also trained in Internal Medicine, have to be careful to speak of "urination," lest we be confused with urologists.

Stuffed comfortably in my mother's womb, I couldn't imagine why there was such a rush to make urine. My mom's kidneys were doing a dandy job of excreting the wastes my body was producing. I was safely connected to her blood supply through the placenta, a marvelous, disposable dialysis machine that lets waste products produced in my body diffuse into her blood to be eliminated in the urine she excreted. Her kidneys evidently sensed that I would be hanging around because they increased their cleansing functions long before the stuff I would be adding amounted to anything. The same thing happens when you donate a kidney to another person. Both kidneys "man-up" and work doubly hard to carry the load in the donor and in the recipient. Nice things, these kidneys. They look out for one another.

You might be wondering what happened to that urine I squirted into the amniotic cavity that surrounded me while I was in the womb. Well, it may sound crude, so get used to it if you intend to continue reading this story. I repeated that exercise over and over, making increasingly larger volumes, literally urinating all over myself for the next six months. And that wasn't bad behavior on my part or masochistic. It was essential. Nature does some surprising things that cultured societies do not always understand or care to know about. Bathing oneself in urine during gestation may be at the top of the list of disgusting acts to be shielded from public awareness.

Failure of an expectant mother to notice that her "waters had broken" during labor or for the physician or mid-wife to find no drainage when the "bag of waters" is incised prior to delivery are ominous signs that the baby will likely die shortly after birth, not because the kidneys need to remove waste products from the blood — the mother's kidneys have taken care of that — but because the kidneys have other essential tasks to perform in fetal development. The urine I passed into the amniotic sac helped to fill the space between me and the wall of my mother's uterus, thus providing me with a protective "bumper" that prevented any bruises when mother did her laundry or vigorously bowled several frames and slammed me against a bowling ball. Babies with congenitally missing or obstructed kidneys make no urine and consequently have a scant amount of that protective amniotic fluid (*scant amniotic fluid = oligohydramnios*). Unfortunately, these babies die before or shortly after birth.

Now you'd better be sitting down before you read on. I drank the amniotic fluid containing my urine to practice swallowing before I had a real nipple to suckle. I also inhaled the amniotic fluid into my water-logged lungs in order to bathe them with growth factors excreted in the urine that were needed to make my lungs mature properly. That is why babies born without kidneys also have poorly developed lungs that ineffectively absorb oxygen from the air shortly after birth. So you see, the kidneys are essential organs before as well as after we are born. Perhaps urine won't seem so disgusting to readers who accept the fact that they, too, bathed in it, drank it and inhaled it for several months before adapting to a terrestrial lifestyle.

Despite the fact that kidneys are a vitally important source of the "birth waters," their role is not mentioned nor is urine included in the rituals of any religion I know of. Most Christians are brought into the faith through a ritual of baptism, patterned after the episode in the book of Matthew reporting how John the Baptist dunked Jesus in the Jordan River to symbolize that his cousin had been "born again" (John 3:3-8). Now that the biologic facts about fetal development are more widely known, it would add authenticity to a sacred ritual, especially for those who take biblical teachings literally, were a few ounces of the initiate's urine added to the water in the baptismal fount.

Dr. Logan Dennis had to clasp my head between two stainless steel blades he had inserted into the womb, compress the forceps together and then pull with as much force as he could muster. Once my head was out the rest came quickly. Weighing in at 9 pounds 13 ounces, my face and body looked more like meatloaf than pink baby. But I ended up with two fine kidneys and a healthy urinary tract that showed off their combined firepower when my projectile stream of new-born urine hit the cheek of a nurse who was standing beside my mom half-way across the delivery room. After a 48 hour "high forceps" delivery, I had earned the right to attack my tormentors when released from confinement. It took more than 50 stitches to repair the damage I did to my poor, exhausted mother during my passage through her birth canal. Interesting how she would cannily find a reason to replay the horrors of my birth whenever she wanted me to do something against my will. My sister, Annetta, came along 14 years later. Her birth had little drama as she weighed only 6 pounds and she didn't pee on anyone in the delivery room.

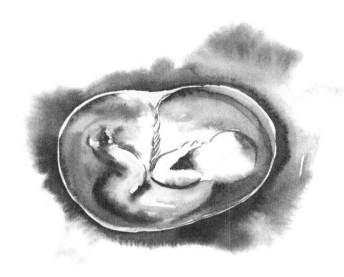

CHAPTER 2

Solutions around the pickle barrel

It must have been the time I spent immersed in amniotic fluid that stimulated my interest in water, for I was born into a land so crispy dry that gunfights once decided whom the water rights belonged to.

My father, Jimmie, was born and raised in Dodge City, Kansas, the frontier town of "Boot Hill" fame. Shortly after his birth, his dad (my grandfather) took off to find his fortune in the far West leaving the family with no means of support. Relatives suspect he left because my grandmother had found another lover, and indeed, shortly after her abandonment she moved in with Mr. James Hall, a painter and wallpaper-hanger with a decent source of income. My infant father was out-sourced to a family friend and my grandmother gave birth to three more half-siblings before he could rejoin his family. Despite his initial expatriate status,

5

my father adored his mother and stepfather and had a generally happy childhood until his freshman year in high school. A small but deceptively strong man, he wanted to play football, but his stepfather would not permit it. So my father quit school and went to work "jerking sodas" at Gwinner's Restaurant in downtown Dodge City.

Around 1934, he met my mother, Ista Iola Taylor, when he delivered Cokes and ice-cream sundaes to the beauty shop where she worked as a hair dresser. There he encountered a beautiful woman with dark hair framing a "Loretta Young" face complemented by a hint of Native American or African-American type pigment that harmonized with lips glistening bright red and cheeks tinted with a light coating of rouge. My father was thunder struck by love at first sight.

Born on a cotton farm near Keystone, Oklahoma, now beneath the waters of Keystone Lake on the Arkansas River, my mother finished the eighth grade and longed to go to high school. It was the custom on small farms for children of this age to drop out of school and work full time in the fields. It was a hard life made worse by devastating tornadoes, accidents and illness. Her parents were "share-croppers," tenants who farmed the land while giving the landowner a relatively large chunk of the revenues. The "Okies" described in John Steinbeck's classic novel, "The Grapes of Wrath," captured the situation my mother found herself in. She had enough to eat and clothes on her back, but those were her only tangible assets. She feared her father and adored her mother and her siblings, especially older brother Everett, who had left the farm to work in Tulsa, earning enough money to become a certified cosmetologist. My mother was the most headstrong of her female siblings and she, too, escaped the farm at age 15, lied about her age and got a job at Kresge's Five and Dime, earning enough money to go to beauty school. After graduation and with certificate in hand, she moved to Dodge City, Kansas, where Everett had opened a thriving beauty shop. He offered to hire her for the princely sum of $20 a week plus tips.

My mother had the energy of three persons and could always find something that needed to be done, a trait that would put her in conflict with other ordinary humans in the years to come. Frenetically tidy about her appearance in public, she became a talented seamstress who fashioned feed sacks and discarded material into clothing that would rival the finest store-bought items on Main Street. With hair, yarn, cloth or rocks from Bear Creek in her hands, she could shape, knit, crochet, sew and paint three-dimensional masterpieces with the certainty of an artisan. She had a remarkable memory and was nearly unbeatable in contract bridge and poker. She always came home from the horse and dog races in Raton, New Mexico, with more money than she took. She was shy and usually stood in the shadows at public gatherings. Although polite by nature and careful to use grammatically correct speech, she could transform into an animated, biting, expletive-laden avenger faster than a caped crusader if she believed someone was unfair or trying to take advantage. She won most arguments, earning a reputation as someone you wanted on your team. I have often thought that with a high school education, she might have become the first female chairman of General Motors.

My father was on the other end of the bell-shaped curve, a care-free, happy-go-lucky chap with more friends than he could count. He had a job paying $15 a week, enough money for a bachelor to live the "good" life in Dodge City — until he met and fell in love with my mother. She was rather frosty in social settings in contrast to his unabashed conviviality. But like opposite poles of a battery, when these two loaded up with a couple of high-balls and raced onto the dance floor, sparks spewed out and inhibitions were deferred until the small hours of the morning. They were married in 1934. I interrupted their party in 1936.

We lived in Dodge City for five years. My father found a better job with Fairmont's Dairy delivering milk, bringing with it opportunities for expanded social contacts. I think he and his kin may have invented social networking. The MacDowell reunion, featuring my grandmother's pathologically tribal MacDowell family of Scotch descent, was the "can't miss" event for my father each Memorial Day. It was with this group I learned, in retrospect, of the powerful bonding of human DNA. Dozens and dozens of brothers, sisters, aunts, uncles, cousins, second cousins and cousins once or twice removed gathered at the park in Dodge City along the Arkansas River to eat, greet and brag about the clan's achievements. This was my father's heaven and my mother's hell. Jimmie was a favorite, but there were deep-seated reservations about this "stiff Okie woman" who had captured him. Dad first heard about this chatter from his brother Bob as they gathered around Aunt Madelyn's pickle barrel.

Dad's older sister Madelyn had a secret dill pickle recipe that produced the best pickles in the history of the world. She kept a 55 gallon wood-staved barrel in her basement, and it was timed to produce ripe pickles on Memorial Day. In the Dodge City of that time, pickles and Jim Beam bourbon were as complementary as today's cigars and Scotch whiskey. Kansas was a dry state, so any alcohol in Dodge City had to travel more than a hundred miles or be made locally. Several bottles of Jim Beam always seemed to appear on schedule, usually with a Colorado tax stamp around the cap. The picnic adjourned to Madelyn's basement, and the pickle barrel was ceremoniously opened with a crowbar.

Jim Beam, drunk straight from the bottle and a mandatory "YEEEEHHHH!!" shouted by the beneficiary was followed by the aggressive consumption of a pickle and sometimes chased with beer. Each adult took his turn in the ritual, eventually creating a light-hearted atmosphere in which worn-out, dirty jokes became side-splitting funny and the authenticity of wild tales of male conquest were not questioned. Shortly after this party began, men would begin the trek up the stairs seeking the nearest bathroom for relief. Here I experienced my first tutorial on the diuretic actions of water flavored with barley, hops or sour mash. Cousins judged too young to imbibe the liquid treats felt privileged to witness this complex family ritual, a sort of rite of passage into the MacDowell family adult world.

During one session, the topic of wives entered the discussion (the women were always upstairs or out on the porch and lawn unless they were invited to stand by the pickle barrel). On this occasion, my cousin Sandra and I happened to be standing together in a corner of that sacred room. Most of the comments about the wives were silly or approving until my father's distant cousin mentioned my mother's name in the same sentence with a pejorative descriptor. My father charged the unsuspecting, tipsy fellow, driving him off his feet with a powerful blow to the jaw. Like an atomic chain reaction, the room burst into a saloon fight more vibrant than any staged on the big screen in grade B movies. On that Memorial Day, Sandra and I witnessed the darker side of the MacDowell family reunion that on too many occasions produced an abundance of broken noses, missing teeth, daylong headaches and bruised egos.

When the rumble ended, the small man with the dynamite fists, the friendliest man in town, stood atop a tangled pile of drunken bodies struggling to become upright. All of these men were professed Christians, so before the lid was put back on the pickle barrel and they ascended the stairs to an arcade of scowling spouses, the MacDowell bond was restored with handshakes, hugs and offers of assistance to those too beat-up to walk unaided. Ista was accepted into the family in perpetuity. The messages of the day seemed pretty clear to me at the time: "families that fight together, stay together" and "may God help anyone who insults a member of the family." Viewed in a broader context, the MacDowell clan was fiercely patriotic, and many of the men around that pickle barrel soon took the same fighting spirit to foreign lands on behalf of their Nation.

CHAPTER 3

Discovering water

Fairmont Dairy asked my father to move 70 miles east to Pratt, Kansas, to help start a new satellite business. A town of about 5,000 people, Pratt's economy was supported primarily by farming and oil and gas production. A military air base a few miles north of town had just been completed to train pilots who would later make bombing runs in Europe and the Far East. We rented a house on Pearl Street, a 9-block walk to the elementary school where I began the first grade. We did not own an automobile, but my father had periodic access to a milk delivery truck he would use to run errands for Mother.

My mother was raised in a patriarchal family that attended the Church of God for services twice each week. The Bible was the infallible word of God. Women were deferential to men and wore simple dresses and no make-up. Theirs was a disciplined lifestyle, yet Christian principles also ruled the church and they cheerfully welcomed strangers, fed the downtrodden and came to the aid of neighbors. When my mother moved away from her homeland, she took the Christian principles with her but left the strict discipline behind. She dressed as stylishly as she could afford, painted her face, drank whiskey and beer, danced with men and smoked Raleigh 903 cigarettes.

My parents believed that I needed to learn how to be a Christian, so

I was enrolled in Sunday school at the First Methodist Church. At the conclusion of the first year, I received a certificate of perfect attendance and my own Bible that I was unable to read. I adored my Sunday school teacher who introduced me to the stories in the Bible and to Jesus in particular. She was so convincing that I believed for many years that Jonah was eaten by a whale and that Noah survived the great flood. I asked her if she talked to God or Jesus. I don't remember her exact answer, but I think she cleverly dodged the question while leaving me satisfied that she had something special going on with the deity.

In Pratt, my entrepreneurial mother opened her first beauty shop in a front room of the house and quickly attracted a large clientele. I was allowed to sit in her beauty shop on days when I was not in school and listen to her banter with the customers. I soon became aware that beauty operators have a very special role in the lives of other women, built on an unspoken code of trust. You see, beauty operators are modern incarnations of the Oracle of Delphi and serve as uncertified marital counselors. Intelligent women will confess everything on their minds to someone who repeatedly and carefully uses hands to clean, caress and sculpt hair. My mother was the Michelangelo of hair, a talent that gave her license to the inner secrets of a great number of women over her lifetime. I should think the CIA would have discovered this fundamental truth by now and would have established a national network of informants as powerful as the World Wide Web.

We had more money than ever. Nonetheless, my multitasking mother thought we should raise chickens because meat was expensive and hard to find with the war going on. My job was to feed and water the chickens and gather the eggs. As if it needs to be taught, I was learning the importance of drinking water for sustaining life.

Pratt had a slightly wetter clime than Dodge City, and grass would grow for most of the summer without adding extra water. Having no automobile, we relied on taxis for important trips or we walked. I discovered a huge municipal swimming pool two miles east of my home where my father taught me to swim. I spent most summer days at the pool turning into a person of color while celebrating the buoyancy of water.

Something about that aquatic experience apparently increased my thirst for water throughout the day. One thing easy to learn about renal function is that a lot of what is drunk by the mouth comes out through the kidneys. During this stage of maturation, my distended urinary bladder would forcefully alert me to find the bathroom in the early morning hours before dawn, and on command, I would arise while in a deep sleep and begin the trip on instinct. On several occasions, I stopped short of the bathroom. Once I filled the glass-bottomed cover over the coffee table in the living room. My mother had acquired this stylish piece by saving Raleigh 903 cigarette coupons. Had I been our pet dog, she would have rubbed my nose in the urine to break any tendency to repeat the sacrilege. Sometimes I ended up in the closet of my parents' bedroom, filling one of my father's boots. After consultation with our doctor, the somnambulism was cured by withholding oral fluids after 6 pm each day, another home-taught lesson in practical renal physiology.

The prominent role water seemed to be playing in my life included my father taking me fishing at Pratt Lake. We would stake out a position on one of the boat docks, load our hooks with rank smelling chicken entrails or shrimp bait and heave our lines into the water. We seldom caught anything, but we would sit there and share our dreams until late at night when dive-bombing mosquitoes would convince us to leave. In the more bucolic moments, I developed a deeper appreciation of and affection for my father and his unrequited dreams he hoped to see played out in my life to come. I think it is fair to say that water bonded us for life.

My mother, on the other hand, had other dreams for me. I was enrolled in dancing lessons shortly after we moved to Pratt. Within five months, I was dressed up in red, white and blue satin pants, a jacket and a top hat, tapping in a recital to the tune of "Yankee Doodle." At five years of age, I knew the difference between my left and right foot, but unfortunately, they seemed to want to move in strange directions under my command. Mother reluctantly averred that I would not be the next Fred Astair.

Undeterred, she set me up to take piano lessons from Mrs. Mert Newhouse whose studio was conveniently located on the street I walked along on my way to school. I remember the little, cream-colored, marble busts of Mozart and Beethoven sitting atop her studio piano, leering at me during the lessons. On several occasions, I am convinced that I saw a tear run down the cheek of one or both of them as I stumbled through one of their adaptations for beginners.

There was one assignment named "Poem" that I thought I had mastered in my fourth year at the piano. It was a masculine piece that I played triple fortissimo. I memorized it in time for Mrs. Newhouse's annual student re-cital held in the cavernous performance hall of the high school. Students who participated were rewarded with a shiny nickel from Mrs. Newhouse as they walked off the stage, enough to buy an ice cream cone. My turn came, and with bombast and arms flying into the air, I super-charged the first half of "Poem" to perfection. My prideful parents struggled to remain in their seats, and a friend told me that Mrs. Newhouse even smiled! Then disaster struck. My mind went blank. There was no oxygen in the room. My hands dropped to my side; I got up, bowed and walked off of the stage to strong applause. Most in the audience, there to hear their own children perform, clapped loudly in ignorance. My parents were gap-mouthed, and Mrs. Newhouse held onto the nickel. With the equivalent of five thumbs on each hand and an undependable memory, I finally persuaded my mother to give up after five years, finishing my piano career stuck in John Thompson's third grade book.

There are hundreds of events that affect our extended journeys along life's path, some more momentous than others. In my case, several of these "shaping experiences" were near misses, where a slight change in timing or position could have finished my life story before I got to the logical ending.

My father always planted a garden with high hopes that we would be covered in abundance. There was a large, vacant lot behind our house that he had plowed in the early spring. An African-American man with a horse that pulled a large steel blade came by each year and turned the soil of the garden patch. It was entertaining to watch this process, and on one occasion, several of my playmates gathered with me to take it in, at least for a while. We soon became bored with the repetition and started chasing one another across the fresh-plowed earth, stumbling and falling, frequently. One of my girlfriends took after me, and I escaped into the street while looking back at her. But just as I turned my head, I ran directly into the side of a van that was moving along at a reasonable speed. The left rear tire ran over the toes of my right foot as my forehead crashed into the side of the truck. I was ejected backwards, crashing onto the pavement in a heap.

My mother heard the commotion and came running out of her beauty shop to my aid, shrieking all the way. A lump the size of an egg had risen on my forehead, and my right shoe had been shorn in half, exposing my bloody bare foot with the nail dangling perilously from my right great toe. My injury looked worse than it turned out to be. I was fully conscious with a frontal headache and a right great toe that felt like it was ablaze. My mother regained her composure and asked the driver of the truck, who was shaking worse than my mother, to take us to the doctor's office as there was no hospital in Pratt. The doctor washed my foot with stinging water and in a flourish pulled the loose toenail from its last connection to my great toe. I learned there that the easiest way to avoid protracted pain was to solve the problem as quickly as possible. I was relieved to have the thing removed, but my mother suffered a fainting spell as she watched the brutal extirpation. This close call counts as my second shaping experience, the first being my tortuous birth.

CHAPTER 4

Life on the Kansas desert

Cousins Peggy and Doris Carter moved in with us after my mother's sister died of a pulmonary embolism. Their father had wasted no time marrying the quintessential Cinderella stepmother, and my pretty cousins sought refuge with us. I was a male in paradise with two virgins within sight right in my own home. It also gave my mother two additional targets for her insatiable quest for orderliness.

As for my music lesson, my mother decided that I would probably do better with a musical instrument that required playing only one note at a time. She was correct. My violin career began with a flourish, and within a year, I was on my way to the first chair of the New York Philharmonic.

In 1945, my parents bought the house we lived in and their first automobile, a 1932 Plymouth sedan with wooden spoke wheels and mechanical brakes. During the war, American automobile companies made tanks and airplanes. A pre-war automobile that would start and go was a prized possession, even if it was a relic. It took a deftly coordinated series of hand and foot movements to get our car started, and my mother quickly became proficient even in freezing weather. However, she had difficulty keeping the engine running while working the clutch and manual gearshift. On many occasions, a trip to the grocery store became a series of lurches punctuated by mother's shouting war-faring expletives. On one memorable trip home from the store, while driving down a small hill, we saw the left rear tire go rolling on before us. Somehow she managed to get the car home, and I went back and fetched the runaway tire.

Cousin Peggy, whose dresses mother skillfully crafted out of chicken feed sacks, was friends with several girls in junior high school whose fathers were lions of industry in Pratt. Now that our family had "wheels," on rainy or snowy days, Mother would treat us with a ride home from school, except for Peggy who did not want her friends to see her get into a movable car wreck. She got no sympathy from the rest of us when she arrived home drenched or frozen to the core after walking 9 blocks facing a harsh Kansas wind.

My parents' big moment arrived in 1947 when my father was offered the opportunity to become a managing partner of a new furniture store in Johnson City, Kansas, about 150 miles west of Pratt. Our home in Pratt was sold for cash, and my father bought a 1940 Chevrolet pickup truck and drove to Johnson City to remodel and open his new store. The rest of us stayed in Pratt to organize our furniture and other possessions for the move west. Leaving Pratt was not easy for me. I cried when we sold mother's old washing machine, the one I nearly ruined when I stuck a toy gun in the wringer.

We finally said all our goodbyes in Pratt and set out for Johnson City with my mother driving the Plymouth and my father the Chevrolet pickup, both vehicles overflowing with household goods, clothing, furniture and pets. We looked only slightly more prosperous than the "Okies."

Our new hometown was situated in one of the flattest places on Earth. In Johnson City, the wind never ceases. In good years, Johnson City receives about 10 inches of rainfall, leaving pastures and lawns brown except for a few precious days following a thunderstorm. Most of the land surface is plowed and planted with wheat, corn or milo. In "wet" years, the crops flourished and people were well off, but dry years brought reduced incomes and unrelenting dust blown off of the barren fields to find its way into every niche and fissure of a home or business.

Fortunately, when we pulled into town, the harvest had over-filled the grain elevators and golden wheat was piled in long rows unprotected from the elements. With such abundance, everyone was happy and ready to buy new furniture. My father had rented a derelict building that had been built around the turn of the century and had lain abandoned for nearly 15 years. A simple, oblong, two-story structure, the floors were connected by a steep interior stairway made of steps about 5 inches wide. You either paid close attention going up and down the stairs or you damaged a body part. The furniture store was on the ground floor and the living quarters were upstairs.

My father had done a respectable job renovating the store on the first level and filling it with merchandise. Business was flourishing, and he was having the time of his life making new friends of each customer that walked through the front door. The upstairs living quarters were another matter. Dirt blown into the building for many years had filled the cracks between the boards in the floor. On our hands and knees, we dug the dirt out of every crack with screwdrivers until mother was satisfied, and satisfying her proved to be the hardest task of all.

Sewage presented another problem because Johnson had no sewer system, and homes and businesses relied on septic tanks or outhouses for disposal. We had an outhouse behind the store, meaning we had to walk down the daunting stairway and go out of doors about 50 feet to use the "two-holer" available to us. To circumvent such frequent trips for liquid waste, my father had purchased a chemical toilet for the upstairs bathroom that was to be used only if someone was unable to negotiate the adventure trail to the outhouse. Being stout for my age, I was nominated as the person in charge of carrying the refuse that accumulated in the chemical toilet to the privy. I sometimes wonder how I developed my interest and affection for urine considering how I hated that detail.

Once we settled in, I explored the neighborhood for new friends and found one directly across the alley behind the store. Ronnie Wilkerson, a year older than me, had lived in Johnson all of his life and was eager to educate me about boy's life on the high plains. There were no television sets, video games or cell phones so we made our own entertainment. Ronnie's father subscribed to "Popular Science" magazine, which we devoured together each month. In one issue, design features of a telegraph system were presented, and from raw materials, we built two senders and receivers, which we connected through a car battery and about 30 feet of wire to our respective outhouses along the back alley. We took advantage of our membership in Boy Scouts to learn the Morse Code. We would sit for hours in our respective out houses in oppressive heat or body-numbing cold to exchange bits of information about much of nothing. Come to think of it, we were years ahead of our text-messaging, time-wasting grandchildren.

Ronnie and I traded comic books on a regular basis. We would usually sit on the kitchen floor in our mothers' way and argue about how many Plastic Mans were worth one Superman. During one of these settings, Ronnie was unusually quiet and appeared sad. Then, without notice he blurted out, "I have polycystic kidneys. And my mom's got them, and my grandma had them."

I don't remember exactly what I said, but I can imagine it was something like, "Huh? What's that?"

He tried to explain that his kidneys were full of water sacs or something like that. I was in the 6th grade and not attuned to or much interested in medical problems. Carrying that chemical toilet down those creepy stairs had buried, for the time being, any latent interest in kidneys or urine. I can imagine that I said something like, "I'll give you a Superman for two Archie's." Years later, it occurred to me that he had spoken of his grandmother in the past tense. He had just returned from her funeral and probably learned at that family gathering that he had a kidney problem that one day would take his life. The topic of Ronnie's cystic kidneys didn't come up again for several years.

I seemed to have more time for dreaming in this desolate landscape of western Kansas, there being no streams or lakes to fish in and the nearest swimming pool 5 miles farther west in Manter. My father had purchased a heavily used typewriter with key faces that had never been cleaned. It was difficult to differentiate an "a" from an "e" as the respective keys only printed a smudge. Nonetheless, I diligently crafted my first novel pecking at the keys with my right index finger. Out poured "Homer: A Poor Man's Dog." I cannot recall why I named the dog Homer, but this prescient name will surface several times in the pages to come. Incidentally, the novel never made the best-seller list.

There were no violin teachers in Johnson or any nearby towns so I took up the trombone, another one-note-at-a-time instrument within my skill level. I found the trombone fun and relatively easy to play. My parents' good friend and former high school music teacher, Gwen Plummer, also discovered that I had a decent singing voice, inheriting "singing genes" from my tenor father and contralto mother. Gwen recruited me to sing tenor (until my voice changed) in the Methodist Church. My boy-soprano days ended in the eighth grade, and I sank to the more common baritone register, although my range was high enough that I was "pulled" into the tenor section frequently for supplemental support.

One day, Mother announced that she was pregnant. She had had one miscarriage after I was born, so she and my father were ecstatic. Dr. Ross Fields, the family physician, instructed her to stay in bed or in a chair for at least three months, meaning that Peggy, Doris and I had to pitch in and do more. It also meant that Mother could no longer make the descent to the outhouse, and that I would be making more hazardous trips with the big bucket.

After three years living above the store on Main Street, we moved into a three-bedroom, two-story house near the edge of town. Peggy graduated from high school and moved back to Sand Springs, Oklahoma, to be nearer to her brother, Bob, and other aunts and uncles. I think she also needed relief from my mother's never ending "suggestions" for self-improvement. Doris stayed behind, intent on finishing high school in Johnson City while also seeking perfection in my mother's eyes.

Ronnie was a freshman in high school and I was in the eighth grade on a separate campus, so we saw less of each other. Donnie Richard and

I had been pals since the sixth grade, and we became especially close as basketball teammates in the eighth grade. Our team unexpectedly won the Syracuse tournament and finished the season with a strong winning record, forecasting even bigger triumphs to come in high school. Donnie also had a car to drive to school from his farm home east of town. The summer before high school was one of the hottest on record. I worked at odd jobs and found any excuse I could to hitch a ride with Donnie 5 miles to Manter where a public swimming pool was waiting just for us.

The Manter pool was filled at the beginning of summer and drained when school began in the fall. There was no filtration system, so the accumulation of dirt blown in by the wind and the outer layers of skin and other refuse from hundreds of bathers produced, by mid-July, a turbid liquid that hid persons swimming 2 feet underwater. Evidently, the germ theory of disease was unknown to the good people of Manter.

I enjoyed diving head first into the water from the 4-foot board. My last dive into the Manter pool set up my third "shaping experience" as my head struck the flank of an invisible swimmer gliding silently beneath me, snapping my head back and leaving me unable to move for at least a minute. I felt like a human tuning fork. Donnie saw what had happened, swam to me and calmly helped me to get out and sit on the edge of the pool where I regained my senses and the use of my extremities. My neck hurt fiercely, and I couldn't turn my head to either side without accentuating the pain. Donnie got me to his car, drove at warp speed back to Johnson City and hauled me into Doctor Fields' office where I was examined and x-rays were taken. There was no fracture, just a severe strain. Doctor Fields thought that with rest and gentle exercise, my neck and the rest of me would probably be ready to start football practice within the month. That news was a great relief as I did not want to disappoint my father, who believed that my 6 foot 1 inch, 198 pound frame insured that someday I would be inducted into the Football Hall of Fame, a goal that he was denied. My next major challenge was to go home and face mother.

❖

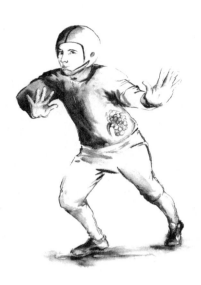

CHAPTER 5

A change in plan

I survived the swimming pool injury and my mother's rage. A few weeks later, I enrolled in high school with 14 other freshmen students. Professor Gene Reid was the new high school principal and his son Jack was in my class. Five of the freshman boys signed up for football and began the tortuous practices in 90+ degree heat with humidity hovering, thankfully, around 3 percent. Donnie Richard and Eugene Shore's parents would not give them permission to play football. I endured the horrible muscle pains that accompanied running wind sprints until your body would no longer move. Gradually, I began to convert the baby fat into a more muscular frame.

We settled into the high school routine and all was going well. Coach Mont Elliott, who spent most of his time shrieking at the players, exhorting them to super-human performance, evidently thought I showed promise for a freshman so I got to run plays with the first team from time to time. I played guard on the line, and working out with the first team meant that I played next to my friend Ronnie, the comic book wizard, who was the starting center. At the conclusion of practice on one typically hot afternoon, the players returned to the locker room to shower and dress as usual. I stopped by the latrine to urinate and found that I was standing next to Ronnie. As I looked into the latrine, I was shocked to see a stream of bright red urine coming towards the drain — and it was Ronnie's urine. Aghast, I stopped in midstream and asked him what in the devil was going on.

"It's just one of those cysts, Jared," he replied calmly. "I took a pretty hard shot in practice. Happens all the time. Don't worry, I'll drink a lot of water tonight and it'll stop."

I don't remember what I said in reply, as I was still stunned at the sight of seeing so much blood coming out of my friend. With his assurance that everything would be okay, I finished what I had set out to do, showered, dressed and went home without speaking to anyone.

We all have certain visual images imprinted within our memories, and Ronnie's blood-laden urine will be one of the last to fade from mine. That episode at the urinal finds its way into my consciousness frequently, and strangely, not with foreboding but with gratefulness that I was there to observe it firsthand; more about that later.

Mother gave birth to my sister Ista Annetta in September, and at age 14, I finally had some competition. Now I had to grow up. She was a beautiful, healthy baby with a scant amount of blond hair that would one day reach her waist in flowing tresses that the ever-present wind would billow like ripe wheat. That said, I must confess that I paid little attention to her as I was self-absorbed, enjoying the excitement of high school and the adventure of becoming a sport jock.

School and football pushed into October, and I felt good about both. Donnie had a birthday party at his home and invited me and several other classmates to a cook out on his farm. I was the only one who spent the night with him. I've tried hard to reconstruct that, our last time together as students and school friends, but I can't think of anything we did or unusual places that we went that afternoon and evening. About 10 days later, I felt sluggish on the football field, and Coach Elliott spent most of the practice yelling at me.

"What's wrong with you, Grantham, you've got lead in your ass!"

I managed to finish the practice and shower. I had a chill as I was dressing and began to perspire. I seemed exceptionally weak. I hitched a ride home and went straight to bed explaining to my mother that I had a rough practice and needed a long night's sleep. I woke up in the night with teeth chattering chills and belly cramps. My bedroom was on the second floor up a steep flight of stairs. I felt too weak to go down the steps by myself so I yelled repeatedly, with diminishing force, for my father, who always slept deeply. He finally came to my rescue in time to get me downstairs to the toilet where my bowels exploded into the stool. I felt wretched.

Mother thought I probably had the flu and gave me some aspirin and a drink of water. My father carried me upstairs to my bed and piled on more covers. I spent a fitful night chilling, sweating and having innumerable, vivid dreams of people so real that they must have been hallucinations. When morning finally dawned, I tried to get out of bed only to discover that I could not raise my head off of the pillow and that the effort led to excruciating pains in the back of my head and neck. When I reached up to grasp my head, I could not lift my right arm, although I could still lift a wobbly left arm. Something was terribly awry! I screamed for my father and mother who came to my room in a rush. They could see that I was soaked in sweat. I had fouled the bed clothes with feces. I don't remember what they said, but mother held my head against her chest and my father ran downstairs and telephoned Dr. Fields who arrived in my bedroom in less than an hour.

Dr. Fields calmly examined me and then explained to my parents that he would have to do a spinal tap to rule out meningitis. He had come prepared for this procedure based on what my father had told him in their brief telephone conversation. He turned me on my side in a knee-chest position, inserted the needle into my spinal canal and then measured the spinal fluid pressure, which was elevated well above normal. He took samples of the fluid for laboratory examination and removed the needle. He pulled my parents aside to tell them that he was convinced that I had acute poliomyelitis. My parents winced at the news for they were Roosevelt Democrats and knew about polio from the stories they had heard about their beloved leader. My father burst into tears and my mother collapsed into Dr. Fields' arms. He did his best to comfort both of them and then headed back to his office to test the spinal fluid for protein and white cells. The findings confirmed his clinical diagnosis.

At that time, prosperous Johnson City was home to a chapter of the Flying Farmers of America and counted more privately-owned aircraft per capita than any city in America. Dr. Fields telephoned Paul (Junior) Plummer, a young farmer who owned a private airplane, and asked if he could convert two of the seats in his airplane into a bed so he could transport me to St. Francis Hospital, 200 miles east in Wichita, Kansas, as soon as possible. Dr. Fields and Junior met at my home an hour later where the physician explained his plan to my stunned parents and my cousin Doris. Junior would fly me and my father to Wichita where an ambulance would be waiting to take us to the hospital. We needed to move with dispatch because Dr. Fields had detected weakness in my breathing muscles and he feared that at the rate the disease was taking over my body, I might need ventilation assistance, an "iron lung," before much longer.

My parents hurried to gather some necessities my father would need for the trip and the indefinite stay. Mother would remain in Johnson to care for my baby sister and organize their business as best she could. My parents seldom had much cash lying around, but before either of them could fret about how my father would manage alone in Wichita, a wad of 20-dollar bills appeared on the kitchen table from a source that remains anonymous to this day. This was just the first of many times my family would be beneficiaries of the unbridled generosity that permeated this dusty little village.

The trip to Wichita was uneventful and, as promised, an ambulance was waiting to take us to the hospital. My father remained at my side until Agatha Rasmussen, the head nurse on the polio floor, ran him off to find a boarding house and get something to eat. I continued to have fevers of more than 105 degrees, sweats and vivid hallucinations. My right arm was limp, but I could still lift my left arm off the bed. They tested my ability to blow out a match every few hours, and I failed consistently. I was told later that they had parked an iron lung outside the door of my room as a precautionary step. They had no oximeters or blood gas analyzers in those days. Deciding when to move a patient into the tank respirator required great clinical judgment.

The polio viruses also feast in and on the gastrointestinal system, so one of the side effects was the frequent production of voluminous quantities of foul, liquid stool. On one occasion when I was reasonably conscious, a nurse's aide came to clean me up after I had spent the better part of an hour lying on a bed pan. Recall that my mother was a clean freak about one's "body," that part of the backside where solid waste makes its exit. Her use of the "body" euphemism caused some confusion when I was younger. One day we were to attend a funeral, and she told me we would accompany the cortege to the cemetery where they would bury the body.

"You mean that they cut off his body and bury it?" I asked.

We eventually got that descriptive misfire straightened out, but I became more skeptical of mother's misplaced illustrations and neologisms she dreamed up to avoid using embarrassing words in public.

The aide was a new emigrant from Germany, a "war bride," who spoke little English and had not had Ista's course in how to cleanse a revolting "body" after passing stool. She grabbed a single square of toilet tissue and swiped in across my buttocks while announcing boldly, "You clean!"

"The hell I am!" I bellowed as loud as I could with limited wind-power, driving her from the room in fright. I yelled to the next nurse who entered the room to come to my assistance and found a sympathetic soul who personally cleansed me to an end point that Ista would undoubtedly approve.

❖

CHAPTER 6

Two uncommon boys and a common virus

On the third day in Wichita, my temperature did not rise into the stratosphere, and I had no hallucinations. Or did I? Donnie suddenly appeared at the foot of my bed with his father and mother. My father had gone out for lunch, and I wasn't sure my visitors were real. I must have seemed a little remote when I did not greet them warmly. When I was finally convinced that this was not an intrusive vision, I burst into tears. Lucille Richard leaned over and gently lifted me into her arms as only a mother can do. I finally said something like "I'm so happy to see you. To think you came this far to see me."

Homer Richard, Donnie's father, was a craggy-faced farmer with skin that had been baked into tough leather by the sun; nonetheless, he was a gentle man and he replied in a soft voice, "No Jared, we are delighted to see you, but we had to come for a different reason. Donnie has polio. Thankfully, it seems to be milder than what you have. Dr. Fields thought we needed to take precautions, so we drove down here today to check Donnie into the hospital. You can keep each other company."

Donnie and I made small talk for a few minutes until he was taken to his room. I did not see him again for several weeks. My father kept an eye on Donnie for me, sitting with Homer and Lucille as they watched the voracious polio virus sweep through their son's body, wiping out every anterior horn cell in his spinal column. Within 24 hours, he was placed in the iron lung that had been parked outside my room.

The so-called "iron lung," a life-saving tank respirator, was a simple hollow steel cylinder 8 feet long, about 3 feet in diameter and sealed at one end. Beneath the middle of this ominous steel coffin, a large bellows, driven by a quiet electric motor, was connected to the inside chamber where Donnie rested on a flat, padded cot above the vent. At the other end of the cylinder, Donnie's head stuck out and rested on a platform, a foam rubber collar fitted snuggly around his neck and sealed at the free edge to the steel casing enclosing the rest of his body. His head was outside and his lungs were inside the container. When the bellows descended, creating a partial vacuum within the iron lung, life-sustaining fresh air rushed through his nose and mouth and into his lungs carrying the oxygen he needed to survive. When the bellows rose, the process was reversed: the oxygen replaced by carbon dioxide waste. The machine ran through 15 to 20 cycles per minute depending on how Donnie was feeling and his apparent level of oxygenation judged by skilled medical personnel on the basis of vital signs and the color of his nail beds and lips.

There were several portholes on either side of the respirator where nurses or physicians could thrust their hands through snug sponge rubber collars to examine, position, scratch or inject the patient, or just hold his hand.

The iron lung churned along with a predicable hissing tone and rhythm, comfortably reassuring Donnie that sufficient air was on its way. On the other hand, to those waiting in the room for any sign of progress, the cadence established by the moving parts could be a tortuous reminder, a drum roll of sorts, that their beloved had only a finite number of future breaths.

Sealed in that metal canister and unable to move, Donnie endured the high fevers, the tortuous gastrointestinal attacks and the inability to scratch an itch. We both remained in the acute phase of polio, plagued by spiking fevers, for about 10 days. When the virus finally went into hiding, happiness was a dry bed, sleep without surreal dreams and a bedpan upon request, rather than demanding urgency. Testosterone began to stir once more, and I began to take notice of the young, first-year nursing students, called "plebes," falling in love with nearly all of them.

The polio ward census was about 90 patients, made up mostly of young children and an occasional adult. The year 1950 had been unusually busy with several hundred patients hospitalized for periods lasting a few days to several months. Nurse Rassmussen was a masterful leader who rolled up her sleeves and pitched in wherever a nurse or aide needed assistance. She handled distraught parents with deep caring and skill, cultivating a positive attitude whenever she could. Polio victims came under the care of orthopedic surgeons who made daily rounds with the nursing staff, laying on the hands and giving encouragement to their patients. I remember listening each day for their footsteps and the sound of their distinctive voices as they worked their way down each corridor. Donnie and I had both been assigned to doctors Rombold and Lance who shared responsibility for the daily hospital visits. Dr. Rombold, in his 60s, was matter of fact and authoritative in tone, not one to smile much or crack a joke. Dr. Lance was younger and friskier, as likely to hum or whistle as he was examining me, as he was to tell me a stupid joke. Dr. Lance became my favorite and another role model for my own career in medicine.

When the fever broke and my sense of smell returned, I was puzzled by the musty odor that descended on the polio ward during the week. On Fridays, this aroma even overwhelmed the stultifying smell of fish left too long at dockside, which typified Catholic institutions of the time. I learned the source of the stench one morning when they wheeled what appeared to be a wringer washing machine into the room and proceeded to put sections of thick woolen material into a tank filled with steaming water. The water was heated to just below boiling. An aide would reach into the tank with a pair of large forceps, fish out a piece of cloth, wave it in the air to cool it down, wrap it around a leg or an arm and then overlay a thick plastic wrap to seal in the moisture and the heat.

I had just been introduced to the Sister Kenny treatment for acute polio. Sister Kenny was an uncertified, self-made Australian nurse who treated polio patients based on her hypothesis that heating sick muscles a couple of times daily would passively relax them and ameliorate spasms and contracture. Her intent was to keep the muscles alive until new nerves could grow into them. This kind of common-sense therapy was possible in the days before Institutional Review Boards (IRBs), informed consent or double blind controlled clinical trials. And as polio treatment it really worked, but not without some discomfort.

I had just ended 10 days of unrelenting, bed-soaking fevers, and here I was being wrapped in boiling swaddling clothes for an hour twice each day. More sweating, only this time induced with a purpose. My skin began to smell like the wool cloths. I had become the musty smell. I looked forward to nightfall when the hot tubs of foul water would be emptied and the cool breeze of an open window was allowed to waft across my bed. I was unable to arise from my bed. I was still unable to blow out a candle, but I had beaten the iron lung out of another victim. My father brought me periodic reports on Donnie, who was totally paralyzed but determined that he would walk again.

My mother came to visit and my father returned home. She had pictures of my little sister, but I am ashamed to say that I wasn't too interested in them. A 14-year-old boy with dreams of conquering the world doesn't see very far beyond his own nose when he has just made it through his fourth shaping experience.

CHAPTER 7

Count your blessings

Mother stayed with me in Wichita until she was convinced that I was going to survive. She needed to be home with her new baby, and my father was needed to rescue his failing business, meaning I would be left to wing it alone. It was near the end of October, and plans were made for my parents to bring my baby sister to see me for Thanksgiving.

After nearly a month in the hospital, I was still constrained to lie flat in my bed. For entertainment, I had the Sister Kenny treatments twice a day and a pillow radio for listening to Arthur Godfrey in the morning and the soap operas and super hero broadcasts in the afternoon. In the evening, it was Fibber McGee and Molly, Red Skelton and Bob Hope. My local football hero, Galen Fiss, who would later be all-pro for the Cleveland Browns, brought several of his Kansas University teammates to visit me. That was hog heaven.

I was adopted and ruthlessly teased by the nursing students as-signed to the polio pavilion, falling in love with them all. My deep and enduring respect for the nursing profession stems from the lifesaving kindnesses I received from those saints during the uncertain dark days in the Fall of 1950.

A new treatment was ordered that I had heard about weeks before, but had been too weak or immobile to have. Each morning after the

Sister Kenny packs were administered, I was rolled onto a gurney and taken down several hallways using two or three elevators to get to the destination.

"We're taking you to the Hubbard tank," the orderly said.

"What's that?" I asked.

"It's a big bathtub full of steaming hot water that has hoses blowing air in the water against your body. Sort of a water massage."

"Have you ever been in the tub?" I asked.

"No. But I'd give anything to be there."

"Let's trade places," I pleaded.

He just smiled back and pushed me into a large room that had a huge, key-hole-shaped stainless steel tank with two or three jets pushing air into the water. The thermometer on the tank registered 98 degrees Fahrenheit. "More heat," I thought to myself. "Now that's a new experience — sweating in water."

I rolled from the gurney onto another platform that lifted me up and positioned me above the boiling cauldron. I sank slowly into the tank expecting to be par boiled. I was immersed in water up to my neck on an angle that left my toes about a foot lower than my head. I began to feel short of breath and asked to come out of the water. The orderly had evidently seen this kind of distress before and selectively lowered the level of my feet so they were immersed in 3 feet of water. He also raised the upper portion of my body so that my upper chest cage and shoulders were barely covered. This made breathing easier as my diaphragms, one of which was rendered nonfunctional by the polio, moved paradoxically when I inhaled.

Now fast-forward a decade to a darkened room on the 6th floor of "D Building" in the Kansas University Medical Center (KUMC). I would not understand the basis of my breathing difficulty in the Hubbard tank until a friend and I were horsing around with a fluoroscope machine in my senior year of medical school. Pat McCann, my supervising Resident in Internal Medicine, was learning how to use the fluoroscope, an amazing instrument that when positioned next to a body allowed the observer to see internal organs and bones in the chest and abdominal cavities. McCann needed a living human avatar to practice on, and medical students were always fair game. I remembered looking at my feet through a specialized fluoroscope device at a shoe store in Pratt where my mother could certify that the fit between my toes and the tip of the shoes was optimal. I suspect that I picked up a few thousand rads of ionizing radiation on such occasions until the federal government woke up and banned the general use of that technology for other than medical diagnosis. But here, in a "temple of reason," I was again being exposed to colossal amounts of radiation in a quasi-medical situation.

"Okay, Grantham! Take a deep breath!" my chief resident intoned as he stared at the screen.

"Whao! Whao! Do that again … and again."

"What's going on?" I asked.

"Your left diaphragm is rising and your right is falling when you inspire. Damned if you don't have a paradoxical diaphragm. Man, I've never seen that before. Heck of a find."

"Wait a minute," I thought to myself. "He's talking about me like I was a thing standing here."

"What's going on, damn it! I want to know," I said forcefully as I stepped from behind the fluoroscope screen.

"Sorry, Grantham. I wasn't expecting to see anything, and then I saw colon gas up to your left nipple line, and it rose even higher when you took a deep breath. And your right diaphragm descended as it should. You're living off of one lung, my friend, and its work is being sabotaged by that sick left diaphragm," he explained with more compassion in his voice.

McCann was a squat man of Irish background who, with his wife on Saturday nights, when he wasn't on call, would close up Jimmy's Jigger, a favorite bar one block from the Kansas University Medical Center. Despite his legendary drinking, he was an outstanding physician, hungry to learn everything there was to know about the human condition. His gruff exterior disguised the physician inside who would sacrifice a night's sleep, several meals or a planned vacation for a patient.

We turned the machine off and sat down as he calmly explained what he thought was going on. My left phrenic nerve, which has roots in the fourth cervical nerve in my neck, was not working. In most men, diaphragmatic paralysis is caused by a lung cancer that destroys the phrenic nerve as it loops around the left main stem bronchus, the major breathing tube connecting the left lung to the windpipe. Although I had smoked cigarettes since my junior year in high school, I was much too young to have this kind of cancer, so McCann was struggling to come up with a more esoteric cause. Before he could figure it out, I thought of the answer.

"I had bulbar polio when I was 14 years old, and it affected my breathing so much that I couldn't blow out a candle. I narrowly missed spending the rest of my life in a tank respirator — my good friend died in one — and I now have an explanation for why I can't run very far without getting winded, have more trouble than others with altitude sickness and why I became so uncomfortable the first time I was immersed in the Hubbard tank during treatment for acute polio. Come to think of it, when I stand in water up to my chin, I can barely breathe and have to either float on my back or get out of the pool."

"Grantham, you've just described the classical features of a paradoxical diaphragm," McCann said, continuing with a glint in his eye and the trace of a smile on his face. "I'll buy you a pitcher of beer at Jimmy's Jigger if you'll take off your shirt and let my sophomore physical diagnosis class examine you."

I would have been far worse off than having a little breathing difficulty if I went home full of beer to a wife who made Carrie Nation, the axe-wielding, saloon-busting girl from southern Kansas, look civil. So I volunteered to show off my useless lung to 20 or so sophomores who barely knew which end of a stethoscope to blow into, provided that he would let me use him to demonstrate proper technique for examining the prostate when I reached the status of supervising resident. I've yet to collect my end of the bargain.

In the Hubbard tank, the jets were turned on and a surging flow of water cuddled my body in a restorative massage. I knew immediately why the orderly wanted to take a dip in the tank. The trip to the Hubbard tank became the highlight of each day, giving me an advanced appreciation of the healing power of moving water commonly available today in backyard Jacuzzi-armed hot tubs.

I had not lifted my head off the pillow for five weeks, so I decided one day to rise up and see what was on the street beneath the window next to my bed. I had little arm strength and my abdominal muscles were flabby, so it was a struggle to get myself to a sitting position. Suddenly everything turned black, and when I woke up, the nurses and aides were lifting me off the floor and onto my bed, waiting to scold me until they were certain that I was uninjured. I had plunged onto a bedside commode that had broken the fall leaving me with bumps and bruises that would quickly heal.

Nurse Rassmussen admonished me as she caressed my hair. She promised that they would begin ambulation after Thanksgiving, taking it slow since lying flat for so long had upset my blood pressure regulation to the point that my brain was denied enough oxygen when gravity worked against my heart's capacity to pump blood uphill.

"What is it about these stupid hearts, anyway?" I thought. "My kidneys and guts work fine, but the heart takes a holiday when I really need it." Astronauts are confronted by the same problem when living for long periods of time in zero gravity, but they know what to expect when they come back to earth and have the technology to combat it.

I was looking forward to Thanksgiving because my parents were bringing Annie to see me along with a home-cooked turkey and dressing feast. When the day came, I was loaded onto a gurney and taken to the top floor of the hospital and into a pavilion surrounded by a glass enclosure. It was a bright, sunny November day, and I should have been in top psychological form, but I wasn't. News from Donnie's room that morning had not been good. He had a kidney infection and sores were developing on his hips and pelvic bones. I still could not sit up. And I would not be going home with my folks.

The orderly pushed the gurney towards my parents who rose from their seats, as a look of expectancy, forecast by huge smiles, long missing, revitalized their faces. Mother rushed to my side and placed a wet kiss flush on my mouth as she muttered a greeting I couldn't understand. My father claimed the opposite side and held 2-month-old Annie above my head so I could get a good look at her. He lowered her so that her lips could leave a slobbery imprint on my forehead, then he kissed me on the cheek and told me he loved me. I felt one of mother's hands work its way through my extra-long hair as the visiting trio waited for me to say something.

Annie was a plump little thing with short, golden-blond hair. She had a cherubic smile as she hovered above my head, decorated in a dress outfit of dazzling colors that my mother had undoubtedly made. I studied her as best I could from my default position, raised my head up as much as I could without passing out and then pronounced the eagerly-awaited judgment that shall live in Grantham family infamy: "She isn't very pretty, is she?" Then I plopped my head back onto the gurney.

Oh, if only I had known "Silly Helen" before I made a fool of myself on Thanksgiving Day in 1950. "Silly Helen" is my sister-in-law who finds humor in nearly everything and enlivens conversations when she is in her groove. Because she is pathologically honest she also becomes loonier and hilariously funny under stress. She simply cannot tell a lie. One day, she received a call from her expectant best friend telling her that the baby had arrived early and that she wanted Helen to drop everything and come to the hospital to see the child. Helen rushed to the hospital and entered the room just as her friend was removing the blanket covering the newborn as it lay on its back in a crib. Helen says she lurched back when she saw what had to be the ugliest baby ever born — a small head, bulging eyes and low-set ears covered with cherry-red skin.

Panic spurred Helen's breathing rate and sweat popped out on her forehead as she stood on one foot, and then the other, desperately trying to think of what to say? Her friend smiled expectantly as she leaned toward Helen, awaiting her imminent praise. Finally, Helen blurted out with great joy in her voice, "What a baby!" The new mother heard the excitement but not the words and gave Helen a huge hug prompting her errant pulse and respiratory rates to sink towards normal. Helen's solution to her "ugly baby conundrum" would have been so useful on that regrettable Thanksgiving Day in Wichita.

Once before, I had stopped time with an intemperate pronouncement at a dinner party my father's major business partner had given to welcome our arrival in Johnson City. I was seated with the adults at the table and the conversation after we ate seemed to go on for hours. I tried to sit unobtrusively, but late in the session I tuned into a line of discussion about customers who complain too much, to which I offered my profound wisdom, "Yes, this does get kind of boring," meaning the customers, not the discussants. Oh, how these miscreant pronouns cause trouble. My parents admonished me for insulting them in front of our hosts, then yanked me out of my chair and took me home, deeply embarrassed by what I had said. Years later when I peeked at my father's diary, there was an entry, "Today Jared embarrassed us at Louie Stewart's house after dinner." We had a quiet home for a few days after I blew up dinner. They weren't the spanking kind of parents, but upon reflection, I think my mother's silent grimness was much more painful.

So I had done it again, but this time I was in such pitiful shape they would not dare to yank or hammer me for denigrating their beautiful creation. Why I said such a stupid thing I'll never know, but on that day I broke my parent's hearts, hearts that had been severely tested for many weeks. I suspect that the pain of being left alone in Wichita, a tad of jealousy and situational anhedonia (*absence of joy*) were important factors underlying my rudeness. One constructive outcome did emerge from this cruel blunder. I have spent the rest of my life observing how the ancillaries of major illnesses can overshadow the best intentions of sick people who are fundamentally good at heart, and I have done my best to implement those hard-won insights into the practice of medicine.

The turkey feast my mother had brought to celebrate our grand reunion was eaten quietly with a few perfunctory words and sentences sprinkled between bites and chews. Annie just cooed and spit through it all, oblivious to her big brother's Titanic gaffe. The afternoon came to an end, I went back to my confinement and my family began the 180 mile trek back to Johnson City.

CHAPTER 8

Coming back

Stretching exercises aimed at strengthening my stubborn muscles soon augmented the uplifting daily trips to the Hubbard tank. I learned that in rehabilitation units, there are three classes of health care workers: the saints, the angels and the beasts with smiling faces. The nurses are, for the most part, saintly rescuers and interpreters of the physician's proclamations. The aides flutter angelically around the saints doing the tiniest, but essential things to bring comfort to patients. The therapists — they think up ingenious ways to inflict pain while professing empathy as they twist or yank a reluctant extremity closer to a position of function.

Ruthelma Rombold, Dr. Rombold's sister, was in charge of the Hubbard tank room and the physical therapy that was meted out to the prey after they had been softened up by the hot, wet massage. How nice it would have been to always return to one's room for a snooze, but Ms. Rombold would have none of that. She looked the part of the executioner. Medium build with rounded biceps and calves, straight black hair in a page-boy cut, square jaw, high cheek bones, and thin eyebrows outlining a stern face covered with lily-white skin. At least that's how she first looked to me from a supine position.

Let the fun begin!

Despite the initial fear and foreboding, within a week I was sitting up without fainting, had regained full range of motion in my left arm and hand and had regained the use of my right hand. During the following week, I was standing alone and walking down the parallel bars without assistance. Ms. Rombold had me on a fast-track to significant recovery when I noticed that she had also undergone an amazing transformation into a graceful princess who purred sweet encouragement into my ears whenever I reached a new level of physical achievement.

Donnie remained in his tank respirator, his only view to the outside world through a large mirror positioned directly above where his head protruded out of the respirator through the tight sponge collar. His world was upside down and backward. Now I was able to go to his room every day and stay for long periods. The Kenney packs had been discontinued and I had the run of the floor.

Donnie fought depression with the hope, however unrealistic, that one day he would be free of his confinement and able to return home. I struggled to keep upbeat and encouraging as I witnessed each day, help-lessly, the torments of unchanging posture and the inability to scratch an itch. The polio virus is a cunning persecutor, for it selectively destroys the motor neurons controlling muscle movement while leaving intact the sensory nerves, which detect hot, cold, pain and itching.

Donnie and I reminisced about the great times we had in grade school and as camping partners in Boy Scouts. We slogged through pu-berty together, each informing the other of the new anatomic changes occurring throughout our bodies in league with surprising urges that the older boys helped to clarify. Mrs. Lucile Richard was always in the room to tend to her son, and if she was shocked by what she heard, she kept that to herself.

One story in particular may have tarnished her son's perfection to some degree. In the sixth grade, we began to pick up off-color jokes from older boys. This, coupled with a camping trip to the mountains I made with two uncles and my father, filled our quiver with some pretty nasty stuff. We decided to share our funnies with our friends by writing a dirty joke book, which we highlighted with both of our full names on the title page. One day, I left it on the top of my desk and one of the girls in our sixth grade class found it and gave it to the teacher, Mrs. Richardson. She was shocked and disappointed by our crass behavior and threatened to send us to the principal, Mr. Graves, who once took off his belt and forcefully spanked, in front of the class, a bent-over Bobby Wise for unruly behavior. We were honestly contrite and begged for leniency, pledging to never do such a stupid thing again. Since we were first offenders, and she had usually favored us among the other boys in class, we got off with staying an hour after school for a week reading and memorizing Bible verses. After we finished laughing about this episode, we both agreed that Mr. Graves' strap might have been more expedient. Donnie's mother sat stone-faced without comment.

Attempts were made each day to wean Donnie from his respirator. The tank would be opened and his head freed from the constricting collar for as long as he could tolerate. Although he could not move any muscles in his extremities, neck nor abdomen, he had enough working muscle left in one diaphragm to move a little air into and out of a lung. Two hours was his record time for breathing on his own, but he would turn a dusky blue color before he asked to be put back into his metal cell. Donnie was the fastest runner in my class and would have excelled at track and field in high school were he to have had the opportunity. He could tolerate the pain of long distance running, and it was this quality that drove him to throw his respirator aside for as long as was humanly possible.

As Christmas approached, Mr. Richard bought a new, bright red Chevy coupe and strategically parked it on the street below, directly opposite Donnie's room. The car was centrally framed in Donnie's reversed view of the outside world, and his spirits were transiently lifted as he fantasized driving at warp speed along gravel farm roads, one hand on the steering wheel and the other caressing a frightened girl seeking safety in his arms. Which brings me to a recent movie entitled "The Sessions" in which a polio survivor, paralyzed to the same extent as Donnie, is granted his unrequited wish to "know" a woman in the biblical sense.

Helen Hunt's quintessential portrayal of a professional sex surrogate who conjugates with the paralyzed man while he is disconnected from his respirator, helping him to satisfy one of biology's most powerful desires, was startlingly realistic. Oh, Donnie, how I wish you could have had an equivalent tryst more than 60 years ago.

At last the news came that I had been waiting to hear for 10 weeks. I was going home. A fresh round of x-rays of my shoulders and arms were taken, and I was fitted with "wing-splint" braces for both upper extremities to prevent them from drooping and over-stretching the muscles in my upper shoulders. I was supposed to wear them during waking hours for the indefinite future. The muscles of my upper left arm and shoulder had regained about 80 percent of their former strength, my left hand was completely normal and I had a full range of motion without pain. Things were not as rosy in my dominant arm. I had lost 90 percent of the muscle power in my shoulder and upper arm, and about 50 percent in the muscles that control the hand. My left diaphragm was knocked out and there was atrophy in the major calf muscle of my left leg. I had a gerrymandered body, but thanks to Sister Kenney, I had mobility and I could dress, feed and bathe myself. Compared to the future Donnie faced, I had nothing to complain about. I had survived my fourth shaping experience.

CHAPTER 9

Settling for less

I undressed in the bathroom shortly after returning home. I had not looked at myself in a full-length mirror for 10 weeks and was aghast when I appeared to resemble a refugee from a World War II concentration camp. Eighty pounds had melted away from a frame 6 foot tall that looked as if it had been assembled with discarded body parts. My left leg was half the size of the right, my right shoulder was skeletonized and my right upper arm and forearm were half the size of the left. A neck designed for turkeys thrust my gaunt face forward. I scared myself; the reality reflected in that mirror subjugated the homecoming joy.

There before me was visual evidence that I would never be a star athlete or even a third rate instrumentalist. I was officially a freak, a bundle of imperfections that guys would avoid and girls would find uninteresting. This was not just a pity party in the bathroom, I was bordering on a serious psychological meltdown. Today, a therapist might call it the *forme fruste* of a post-traumatic stress syndrome. I had wept for Donnie many times at night in the quiet of my hospital room. This was the first time I had cried for me.

Having disappeared from the homecoming celebration for longer than expected, my father entered the bathroom to find me sobbing uncontrollably. He said nothing as he moved slowly towards where I stood, and with tears flowing swiftly down both of his cheeks, he embraced me with his powerful arms and kissed me on the cheek. My father was a fearsome fighter when he thought the cause was just, but constraining that seldom-used force was one of the kindest men on earth with a knack for providing succor in difficult situations such as this. I have forgotten how long we may have stood there or what he might have said in those initial moments, but I shall remember for the rest of my life the profound power of his love. His presence alone told me he understood what I had been through and that he was proud to be my father irrespective of my physical condition. His presence had assured me that I would finish healing surrounded by the good people of Johnson City. And I do remember that when he broke his silence it was to say that a large share of those citizens had in fact come to our house to welcome me back. With that I mustered enough inner strength to leave the bathroom and greet my friends.

Life quickly moved into a new routine. I went to school and spoke to each of my teachers about makeup work. Fortunately, I had received rudimentary materials from the school once I was able to sit up in the hospital, so I didn't have to go back to square one. Moreover, Principal Reid had assured my parents that I would be given all the support I needed to complete the freshman year with my class. I continued the physical therapy exercises Ms. Rombold had prescribed and wore the disgusting "wing splints" most of my waking hours. I spent many hours visiting with classmates and Ronnie, and made some new friends along the way. Jack Reid, the principal's son, became a treasured surrogate for Donnie. He was undersized for football but had played on the junior varsity his freshman year, demonstrating mental toughness in spite of two knees that kept flying in opposite directions due to loose ligaments. His knees alone doubled the adhesive tape budget of the athletic department according to Coach Elliott.

I visited my hero, Dr. Fields, when he had a few moments to spare in his busy practice. I think he saw in me a young man with good potential who might be facing an identity crisis, and he had a plan for how to deal with it. One day, he took me into his tiny laboratory where he determined blood counts and performed urinalysis. His last patient that day had been a woman with an acute urinary tract infection, and he had spun her urine in a centrifuge and examined the sediment with his microscope. He showed me how to position the ocular lenses of the microscope so that I could see the individual components of the urine sediment on the slide beneath the objective lens. It was a breathtaking moment, for I could see multitudes of tiny corpuscles resting among a swarm of moving specks dashing wildly around the field of view. Dr. Fields explained that the larger elements were white blood corpuscles, also called pus cells, and the moving objects were motile bacteria, the cause of the infection. He had prescribed a sulfa drug, a medicine to ease the discomfort and had increased the woman's intake of water to stimulate urine flow, expecting the patient to recover fully in a few days. I shall never forget that "Ah Ha!" moment nor the time Dr. Fields caught a grasshopper in his garden, dissected the testicles and showed me motile spermatozoa prancing on a microscope slide. With his simple demonstrations, sandwiched between his busy practice and his own family, he uncovered in me a latent biology interest that would segue into a career in medicine.

In February, Dr. Fields called my parents to tell them that Drs. Lance and Rombold were very concerned about a severe bending (kyphosis) that had developed in my neck, the severity of which they had been debating since my discharge in December 1950. My "turkey neck" was secondary to weak muscles in my neck, and they were concerned that a sudden jolt might damage my spinal cord. They recommended immediate surgery to fuse several of the vertebrae to provide bony protection to the spinal cord. My parents were just getting back on their feet, and we had a semblance of a home life as we enjoyed watching Annie do her "firsts" of everything. Fortunately, the March of Dimes, the Kansas Crippled Children Program and the unbelievable generosity of anonymous donors in Johnson had cleared all doctor and hospital charges in Johnson and Wichita related to my treatment for polio. My parents decided they had no choice but to make that dreaded trip to Wichita once again.

I briefly visited Donnie shortly after we arrived. He was in constant pain requiring narcotics, having developed pressure sores over his hip-bones and the thoracic spine. His parents did their best to be cordial in the face of losing all hope for their son.

My surgery was performed without a problem. Bone from the wing of my left hip (ileum) was used to fuse five cervical vertebrae from C2 to C6. Turning and bending my head would be limited, but I would be able to drive a car and perform nearly all other tasks. When I awoke from the surgery, I was lying flat on my back with my head in a sling attached by a cord drawn over a pulley and bearing a weight below the head of the bed. Both of my legs were similarly attached to weights below the foot of the bed, assuring that my neck would be held in a fixed position under light tension for 10 consecutive days. I was given morphine or Demerol on a routine basis to relieve the operative pain, but this caused an ileus (my bowels stopped functioning) accompanied by terrible abdominal pain requiring the administration of additional drugs to move the bowel gas along. I lay there in a suspended state of animation, subsisting on a liquid diet until the doctors decided my neck was healed enough to put me in a cervical collar for the remainder of the healing period.

The day for my ascension arrived, and my doctors and their assistants removed the weights and the neck sling so that I could sit up in bed. They discussed beforehand that I would have orthostatic hypotension and might faint, but what they had not prepared for was that when they slowly and gently lifted my head, the bedclothes remained fixed to the back of my head. Lying in the same position for 10 days had created a pressure sore (decubitus), and my scalp had literally grown into the thin pad my head was lying on.

The same thing was happening to Donnie's backside upstairs in his iron lung, only on a wholesale basis. The medical staff gently lowered my head and left the room to discuss their next steps. On return, they irrigated the top of my head and pillowcase with warm saline, the scab loosened and they were able to separate the pillowcase from my head. This time, I managed to stay upright without passing out and was too excited with my restored orthodox view of the world to lash out at the medical staff for their incompetent care. I wear the quarter-sized shiny spot on the back of my head, reflecting a mini-shaping experience, as a battle scar reminding me to pay close attention to the little things in patient care that can mean a great deal to the person in the bed.

Before returning home, I paid my last visit to Donnie's room. He knew that I was coming, so he had refused his narcotics in order to be as alert as possible when I arrived. His parents stepped out of the room to talk to my mother and father. In those moments alone, Donnie told me that he knew that he was going to die and that he was trying to be brave about it. I couldn't hold his hand, so I put my left hand on his forehead as we spoke in halting phrases through the tears and sobs. I don't remember everything that was said except that I promised him that I would do my best to live for both of us. With that pledge I said goodbye and left the room to collapse in my father's arms.

CHAPTER 10

The transformation begins

Word reached Johnson a few days before Easter 1951 that Donnie had died peacefully. I had troubling feelings about the news and found it difficult to cry, unlike the last time we were together. I had lost one of my best buddies, and yet I was relieved that he was no longer suffering. Upon reflection, I think this was my first encounter with emotional compartmentalization, a psychological defense mechanism I would hone more finely in my nephrology practice. The tears that were contained immediately after Donnie's death have been vented dozens of times since then. His "compartment" opens, and he jumps into my thoughts when I travel alone and spend the night in a quiet hotel room or walk the quiet paths of a flowery garden in some distant destination.

Johnson City morphed into full-scale mourning, reserved for those known throughout the community. A steady stream of visitors drove to the Richard's farm armed with food and flowers, staying only long enough to express condolences. Homer and Lucille did their best to remain cordial despite being profoundly fatigued and prematurely aged by their ordeal in Wichita. They drew some strength by my presence and in knowing how much Donnie meant to me. Whenever I visited them, I did my best to keep the fun things Donnie and I had done together in the forefront of our conversation while avoiding any replay of the hopelessness of Wichita's St. Francis Hospital. This was my first experience with hardcore grief. Losing a friend turned out to be extraordinarily painful, but nothing compared to the loss of a son, as I would learn firsthand many years later.

My classmates were a great comfort to me after the funeral, redirecting my attention to the tranquil life in Johnson and to the job of completing my freshman year in high school. My neck had healed, I was using my "wing splints" less and less and began to believe that I might have a life after all. I also noticed that I was getting more strength in my left arm and hand as well as in my right hand.

Sensing that my jock career was over and that I had other talents to build on, several people came to my rescue. Dr. Fields asked me if I would be interested in doing light janitorial work in his office, and I jumped at the chance of being near this community icon and my role model. When Mont Elliott heard that I was working for Dr. Fields and interested in science, he invited me to be the high school athletic trainer, meaning I would tend to the players aches and pains and taping needs, and best of all, I would travel with the team. I accepted on impulse before I recalled that his last words to me in October of the preceding year had been: "You've got lead in your ass!"

My circle of close friends grew larger as I tended to the physical needs of athletes in football, basketball and track. Leon Stanton, considered large at 190 pounds and 6 feet tall, was a stand-out offensive tackle in football and forward in basketball. Years earlier, we were acquaintances in Boy Scouts when we were forced to sleep in the same bunk on trains taking us to and from the Jamboree in Valley Forge, PA. Now I taped his ankles and gave him rubdowns, making is easy to get better acquainted. Kenneth Hudgens ran the mile in track and needed a lot of tender loving care as well. Kenneth, Leon and I would later adopt Richard Arnold, another polio survivor, into the "Thursday Night Gang," comprised of two teetotalers (Leon and Richard) and two latent party boys (Kenneth and

Jared). Other than shooting rabbits at night, turning over outhouses on Halloween and stealing a few watermelons, we were upstanding young men who have remained friends for life.

Gwen Plummer, who would later become Aunt Gwen when she married my uncle Dennis Hall after her husband, Warren, had died, decided that I should take voice lessons to build upon the bit of natural baritone talent I had evinced in her church choir after testosterone had ruined my beautiful boy soprano tone. Her intervention turned out to be a Godsend. All along, I had had this portable instrument, usually in pitch and requiring that I only intone one note at a time — and to think that I could have avoided the torment of all those failed attempts to satisfy my mother's desire that I find fame in the entertainment industry. Considering the troubled path she had just walked down, she was satisfied when I sang a solo on Sunday morning or crooned the "old songs" with Gwen accompanying me at the piano before a house full of captive guests. I owe so much to insistent women, my mother in particular. I have learned over many years that singing loudly is a socially acceptable means of relieving tension, as effective as yelling or screaming while shaking one's fist at the heavens. And it has proved to be much less expensive than psychiatric therapy.

The sophomore and junior years of high school were not interrupted by more illness or financial distress for my family and me. I began to take more interest in my beautiful sister with the long blond hair that mother coiffed meticulously. Johnson City made the State of Kansas basketball playoffs in Hutchinson in the spring, a first and huge event for the town. Nearly the entire village migrated to Hutchinson to cheer for the team. I travelled with the players, urging them on, taping their ankles and massaging tense muscles when called upon. The night before the first game, I was so hyped that I could not sleep. I tossed until 2 am, and then knocked on the door of the coach's room to be greeted by Mont Elliott, who had a small bottle in his hand. I was evidently not the first nocturnal visitor, for he simply handed me a white pill then shut the door and returned to bed. I have no idea what he gave me, but a few seconds after I took it I was deeply unconscious.

We won our first game and Arkie Morris, the tallest man on the team at 6 foot 2 inches, had his picture making a basket splattered across the front page above the fold of the Hutchinson News Herald, a newspaper distributed widely throughout western Kansas. Johnson City was instantly famous. However, the news about Johnson City rapidly deteriorated when we heard, while hanging out on the streets of Hutchinson between games, that our beloved Dr. Harold Ross Fields had died of a pulmonary thrombosis after falling through the roof of the Pilgrim Holiness Church where he had been helping with construction. We were stunned and disbelieving that such a thing could happen to this iconic man. I was not ashamed to cry along with several of the team members as we ran to find Coach Elliott at our hotel. Before we got there, the coaches had discussed the possibility of forfeiting the next game and returning home, but on the advice of several of the community leaders, they concluded that Johnson City needed something to lift it up, and so we planned to make a run for the championship.

The team was flat and played poorly. Coach Elliott did not raise his usually screeching voice at turnovers or missed layups, as we were decidedly defeated. We returned home in a solemn procession, and I went straight to Dr. Fields' office to clean it for the last time. Ruth Fields, his widow who lived upstairs, must have heard me come in and found me crying in the laboratory, with my hands clasping Dr. Fields' microscope. She put her arms around me, and we sobbed together for how long, I can't remember. She did tell me in parting that Dr. Fields loved me and had targeted me for a career in medicine, which she had seconded with the prediction that I would return to Johnson City to finish the work that he had begun.

I had a lot of trouble with Dr. Fields' death, as it caused me to question my religious beliefs, which up to then had been orthodox Methodist. Why would a kind and caring God destroy one of his most faithful and productive followers — letting him fall off of a building meant to worship the same big guy in the sky? Previously, I had never questioned Divine providence in respect to my own misfortunes, as I always emerged with enough left over to function in society. Dr. Fields' death, so close to Donnie's, made me wonder why the deity was so darned mean-spirited, so hard on the innocents of this world. I got no help with this conundrum from adults or my pastor as they all came up with some dusty version of this being "God's will" or something equally un-illuminating. I still struggle with this issue, but have found some solace in a philosophy based primarily on what Jesus allegedly said and did more than 2,000 years ago.

In the fall of my senior year in high school, I faced another health challenge, but this time I could not rely on Dr. Fields to solve the problem. I had a high fever, coupled with excruciating headaches that were accentuated when I stood up, coughed, sneezed or strained at stool. My mother thought I had the flu that had been "going around," but after a couple of days in bed, when my urine turned deep orange and the whites of my eyes yellowed, she hustled me to the doctor's office in Ulysses, 20 miles east of Johnson. The physician had practiced in Ulysses for many years, and his office was always overflowing with patients, as he had picked up most of Dr. Fields' clientele as well. Part of this excessive business, I came to learn years later, was due to a restrictive covenant he forced any partner to sign before joining him in practice that precluded the new physician from setting up an independent office within a 50 mile radius of Ulysses. It turns out that was a common practice, not only in Ulysses, but also throughout the United States — and still is. I was shocked when I learned about this sordid business practice many years later because it meant that my professional colleagues, who brandished themselves as caregivers, appeared to care more about their own well-being than that of their patients. Dr. Fields' would not have hesitated to take a chicken or a dozen eggs from a poor dirt farmer in distress in lieu of cash payment and would have never presented a new partner with such a contract.

After a long wait with my head killing me, we saw the doctor. He ordered a blood test to be done in his office and then sent me back to the waiting room to await the results. After another hour or so, we were seen once again. In a very matter of fact way, he told my mother that I had a high white count and he wasn't sure what I had. I had had enough biology and health courses in school to know that high white counts could mean that you have leukemia, so I asked, "Could I have leukemia?"

To which he replied hurriedly, "Yes, I suppose you could."

Then he called his nurse in to make arrangements to have me admitted to the small hospital where further tests would be done. He did not give my mother or me any additional information than that. I was devastated by this fifth shaping experience, thinking that it might be my last. At least I had a chance after polio, but all that I knew about leukemia was that no one survived.

That night, several of my schoolmates learned of my new predicament and came to the hospital to cheer me up. I was in isolation, so they tapped on the ground-floor window of my room that I opened to greet them. Kenneth Hudgens, Jack Reid, Lou Ellis, Keith McGehee, Molly Sosa, Phyllis Carrithers and Nancy Trostle carried on for more than an hour, not letting me take this new problem too seriously. They admonished me to buck up and shake it off as I had always done before.

The next morning, the doctor swept into the room and said that my heterophile titer was "off the wall" and that I had infectious mononucleosis with meningitis and hepatitis. He said it was also called the "kissing disease" because it was a common virus on college campuses where a lot of kissing and little studying went on. As he generated the first smile I had seen on his face, he asked me, "Who have you been kissing, Jared?"

Still angry about his leaving me with a leukemia diagnosis, at least in my mind, for several excruciating hours, I probably just ducked my head and said something like, "No one that I know of." He told me that I could go home and stay there until my headaches cleared and my urine returned to the usual yellow color, and then he scurried out of the room to see his office full of patients. I thought to myself, "If I ever practice medicine, God shoot me down if I should leave a dreadfully sick patient without the comfort of knowing that I cared." Sure, he got the diagnosis in due course and I would mend, but to not sense and act on a patient's obvious distress is unconscionable. Well at least with this shaping experience, I would have one less exotic virus to deal with when I went to college.

CHAPTER 11

More hills to climb

The senior year zinged along, and my parents and I started talking about college. I had made up my mind what I wanted to do for the rest of my life, probably in Johnson City. We still had no physician, so why not grow one of our own. During the school year, I kept busy ministering to the athletes and spent some weekends working at the Collingwood Grain Company storage elevator keeping books. I had worked at the same job during the preceding two summers and got to know Fred Collingwood, the owner of this and several other grain elevators throughout western Kansas. "Conservative businessman" is an understatement to characterize him and his business plan. His elevators were all of the gravity-feed type, meaning that in a unit of four large cylindrical grain-filled columns standing more than a hundred feet high, the floors sloped to a central focus where conveyor belts would hoist the grain into a railroad car sitting nearby or into another of the adjacent columns, a process known as "turning" the grain. The gravity feed cut the cost of moving a bushel of grain by 50 percent because electric power was needed only once for essential transfers in contrast to the more stylish linear models, like those seen in the movie "Picnic." He did not paint the elevators, also saving thousands of dollars, and if you looked at him carefully, you would not know that you were talking to a multi-millionaire, for he resembled a commoner who had just finished plowing a dusty field. His house was ordinary and his children dressed like the rest of us.

There was a filling station at the grain elevator where I worked, and Fred would come there periodically to fill up with gasoline and have the oil changed in his car. Being the junior clerk to Marion Seyb, my boss, and Leon Kilgore, who ran the elevator, Fred was relegated to my care and keeping. I washed his windshield to a spotless shine, removing embedded grasshopper carcasses by the hundreds. He reminded me each time I changed the oil to add an extra quart above the recommended capacity. He had a theory that doing this would preserve the life of the engine. It must have worked because he had been driving the same car for about 10 years. I knew that he "took a shine" to me because Marion told me that Fred once came in for car service while I was out of town, and rather than have him or Leon do the oil change, he decided to wait for me to come back to do the work.

Fred and his wife, Edna, were members of the Methodist Church and through this connection had become acquainted with my parents. When they learned that I was thinking of enrolling at the University of Kansas in Lawrence, Fred and Edna telephoned and offered to take my parents to and from a church gathering one evening. The four of them sat in Fred's car in front of our home for more than an hour discussing my future. Fred was concerned that I would get distracted or lost in the mass of students at KU. They both thought I belonged in a more sheltered environment, for example a school with a Methodist connection. His youngest daughter, Martha, a year older than me, was attending Baker University, a small school 15 miles south of Lawrence, founded by Methodists in1858 and the oldest college in Kansas. An older daughter had graduated from Baker. My parents explained to the Collingwoods that they had looked into Baker, but it was much too expensive for their budget. They could manage the lower tuition at KU if I could obtain a scholarship hall award that included room and board.

They also told the Collingwoods that I was going to have orthopedic surgery on my right shoulder to make it easier for me to lift my right hand above waist level. Polio had severely weakened the biceps and triceps muscles of my upper right arm and all of the shoulder muscles on the same side. Consequently, I could not use my dominant right hand to do anything above the level of my waist. Moreover, when I placed my right hand above a girl's waist at the beginning of a dance, it was a struggle for me to keep it above waist level as I led her around the dance floor in a fox trot. More often than not, my hand would slip down over the soft, fleshy part of my partner's buttocks, earning me a "fresh boy" reputation who couldn't keep his hands to himself. I was overjoyed when Dr. Lance, my orthopedic surgeon hero, staffed a Kansas Crippled Children's clinic in Dodge City and told me that an operation would fix this problem.

Spring came and the senior class at Stanton County Community High School in Johnson City, Kansas, made preparations to finish the year with panache. Nancy Trostle and I were "going steady," meaning we held hands a lot and occasionally snuck off in a car to rehearse the fine art of necking. I was never quite sure what she saw in my deformed body and me. Maybe I was just the last guy in our class who she had not gone out with. Our class took the annual senior trip with 13 students and four sponsors to Corpus Christi, Texas, to swim in the Gulf of Mexico, to travel into Mexico and buy our first bottles of liquor that were clandestinely consumed beyond the awareness of our sponsors. We were experiencing freedom for the first time and fortunately no one was maimed or killed. The only tangible evidence of our collective mischief was the Navy-themed tattoos Duane McGowan and Keith McGehee had drilled into their deltoid muscles surrounding the right shoulder joint. Mr. Reid was not too happy about that, but there was no way to erase the damage. When I last saw these guys at our 50th high school reunion, the tattoos were as vivid as the day they got them.

Following graduation, I headed to Wichita to have the head of my right humerus (upper arm bone) fused to my right scapula (shoulder blade bone). The clever orthopedists had detected preservation of the upper half of my right trapezius and the upper part of my right sternocleidomastoid, muscles used to shrug the shoulder girdle. The upper portions of these muscles are innervated by nerves coming from the medulla oblongata in the head and had been spared injury by polio. By fusing the humerus to the scapula, I would be able to lift my right arm and hand to retrieve objects a few inches above eye level, and I would be able to dance and only caress the buttocks of maidens I sensed would welcome such attention. I would be armed and ready for college.

But first I had to get through the surgery. I woke up in a cast covering my upper body, my right arm raised to nipple level with my elbow bent to 45 degrees and the forearm fixed to the cast covering my abdomen by a one-inch square stick more than a foot long and covered with plaster. Awkward is not an adequate word to describe the sensation. I was on my feet by the second day and ready to go home on the third. This time, none of my body parts stuck to the sheets covering my hospital bed, although I did question Dr. Lance about how I was going to scratch an itch in my back, abdomen or elbow should that undoubtedly happen. He said he heard that girdle stays were quite good for that, but that I should not use wires with sharp points or I would cause damage to my skin. Armed with that valuable knowledge, we went looking for girdle stays several decades after women stopped wearing the ones containing the required length.

I was quarantined to quarters that summer, with an evaporative air cooler to lower the outdoor temperatures of 105 degrees in the shade to approximately 80 inside. We had no television, iPads, computers or tweets to help pass the time, and reading a book with only one hand was a challenge. I listened to the radio and especially to the Liberty Broadcasting System that carried a major league ball game every day of the season. Nancy looked in on me frequently and would take me for a ride in the cool prairie evenings. The body cast put an end to our smooching, but it was nice to have her company. Our respective families believed that one day we would become engaged to be married, but before summer ended, it was clear to both of us that we each had a lot of life ahead and it would be better not to be tied down. She had enrolled in McPherson College where her parents graduated, and I had received a Summerfield scholarship to Kansas University. The Kansas Crippled Children's Program was also kicking in funds for books, supplies and travel to and from college.

The cast was removed in mid-August, and the rather rank odor of two-and-a-half months of accumulated sweat and other detritus went with it. It crossed my mind that my cast may have helped Nancy to decide to explore greener pastures. I was instructed to wear my wing splint for several months and do exercises to extend a contracture that had developed in my right elbow, preventing me from straightening my right arm. When we got home, I hopped into the bathtub and soaked for an hour. My right elbow was severely bent and the skin across the ante-cubital surface was very tight. Later that evening, I asked my cousin Doris, who had come to visit, to help me straighten it out. She was a strong woman and began to extend my arm to ever increasing limits as I yelled expletives at the top of my lungs. She was relentless, and when she reached a point that she wasn't strong enough to make more progress, she sat on my lower arm and pushed against my humerus with all of her might. I feared that she would rip the muscles from their insertions on the bone. Finally, she wore out, and I was taken off the rack. Unfortunately, she was not around to continue this torment for a few more days or I would not have been left with a 15 degree permanent bend in the elbow. Except for this crooked reminder, everything else that Dr. Lance had promised came to pass.

Two weeks before my scheduled travel to Lawrence, Kansas, to enroll in KU, I received word from Mr. Reid that Baker University had awarded me a full scholarship from anonymous donors. Prof's son Jack, with whom I had grown very close during the senior year, was also enrolled at Baker in pre-engineering and had secured a room in Jollife Hall, the only male dormitory on campus. At this late hour, Baker had found a room for me in a private home and was waiting for my response.

I had not been able to visit either campus, so my parents and I had to make this decision on instinct. We knew Richard Arnold and Martha Collingwood would be on the campus of 500 students along with Jack, so having them available to help with the adjustment settled the decision in favor of Baker. I did not learn that the anonymous "donors" were Fred and Edna Collingwood until years later when Mr. Reid told me at the 25th reunion of our high school graduating class. Martha Collingwood was not aware either, but she learned after her father had died that her parents had done much silent philanthropy through the years. Fred's penny-pinching business plan evidently gave him extra money to give out to those who needed it most. The Collingwood's unheralded generosity is a fine model for those who profess to be caring Christians.

CHAPTER 12

The Baker U. metamorphosis

During the last week of August 1954, my grieving parents helped me onto the Santa Fe train to Kansas City, Missouri, during its brief stop in Syracuse, Kansas, 27 miles north of Johnson City. Dad tossed two suitcases into the entranceway leading to the passenger compartment and then waved goodbye along with my mother and Annie as the train jerked forward. My right arm supported in the splint strapped to my upper body made it difficult for me to get two uncooperative suitcases into the passenger compartment through sliding doors that needed three arms to manipulate. When I finally got everything into the passenger compartment, I saw others standing in the aisle — and they weren't just stretching their legs. The train was packed, and there was not an empty seat in sight. I thought that surely my wounded limb would generate some sympathy and a kind soul would offer me a seat. Not on an August day in Kansas with the temperature in excess of 100 degrees Fahrenheit and an evaporative-type cooling system that did little more than raise the humidity to tropical levels.

I stood until we were halfway across Kansas. We stopped briefly many times, but no one moved from his or her seats in my car. Finally, in

Newton a man got up to exit the train, and I was in his seat before it had cooled below body temperature. It was nearly midnight and within seconds I was in a deep sleep known only to teenagers. We passed through Lawrence as the sun was coming up, and I regained consciousness just as the conductor readied everyone for arrival at Kansas City Union Station.

I could see Uncle Roy and Cousin Bob waiting for me rail side. I think Uncle Roy may have smiled as he shook my hand and grabbed both bags while turning to sprint toward the nearest exit. A man of few words and always in a hurry, he led me through the throngs of arriving and departing passengers in the cavernous waiting room and into the parking area near the entrance. Before I could figure out where north was, we were on our way to Baldwin City, 45 miles southwest of Kansas City and about 15 miles south of Lawrence.

Uncle Roy stopped at a filling station in Baldwin City and got directions to my boarding house that turned out to belong to Bill Horn, the son of the Baker president, Nelson Horn. It never occurred to me that living in Bill Horn's house would have anything to do with Fred and Edna Collingwood and Mr. Reid. Years later, I can only imagine the conversation that might have taken place prior to my arrival.

"Gene, Edna and I think that Jared will get lost at KU. He's untested in a man's world and could get in with the wrong crowd as he tries to 'sew his oats.'"

"Yeah, I know him pretty well. He's had the brakes on since he had polio. KU will be the fast lane and he could lose his way. That's why we're sending Jack to Baker. Your girls are wild about Baker and have convinced Leona and me. They have fun and they're doing very well."

"Gene, we're ready to pay Jared's full costs at Baker if that's what it takes to get him there. Do you think you could set that up with the college?"
"I'll call President Horn tomorrow. I met him when we took Jack to look Baker over. He's a reasonable man, and when he learns about the kind of student Jared is, I think he'd be a fool not to take the deal."

Uncle Roy carried my bags to the second floor of the Horn's home to a room on the northwest corner of the building, dropped them in the middle of the room, turned and shook my hand and scurried down the stairs and out the door to his car, immediately tearing off to the highway. I think I told him thank you for what he had done for me that day. My head was in such a spin, and with sleep deprivation, I'm not sure of any detail at the time except that I was tired and powerfully hungry. I did not notice that a room on the northwest corner of the building would guarantee high temperatures in August and September. There were two desks in the room and two chests of drawers.

Looks and clothes had not been high on my list of priorities the past four years in contrast to breathing, gaining strength in my extremities and catching up in school. With the help of some marvelously kind high school teachers, I not only caught up but also earned the Salutatorian title in our class of 13 seniors. The Valedictorian title went to Jimmy Jellison, a preacher's kid who had a math brain and an excellent memory. Jack was really smarter than either of us, but he made a strategic blunder and took a typing class. With gimpy arms, I managed to earn a 50 word per minute typing certificate and an A grade to go with it. Jack may still be taking the test. He typed so slow that the bell would not ring at the end of a carriage run.

I had let my hair grow long during the summer I spent in the body cast and had discovered Brylcream. Hair bathed in this stuff, slicked back with a coarse comb, stayed in place and looked cool — at least no one in Johnson City said otherwise. I wore black, horned-rim glasses that had broken across the nose, requiring tape to keep them on my face. For all I know, I created the "geek look." These fineries together with a pea green seersucker short-sleeved shirt and blue jeans would not set a new fashion trend on the campus.

I washed up, combed my hair and tried to look presentable as I walked downstairs to get better acquainted with my landlords. Bill Horn was a businessman in Baldwin City and was easy to converse with. His wife was sweet and their two children didn't seem to find anything to hate. There were no hard and fast rules of the house except to not behave like caged beasts. My growling stomach kept reminding me I had not eaten for a day, so I asked for directions to the town center and set out to explore Baldwin City and Baker.

The sun had set but the humidity had not. I was used to 1-2 percent humidity; here it was more like 80 to 90 percent. I had not walked a block before sweat began to run down my face, into my eyes and ears and the telltale signs we all hate — wet armpits — blossomed. In Johnson City, the wind never takes a holiday; here there was no air to turn. I found Main Street, which on a Sunday night in any small Kansas town is typically funereal. Deel's Café was open, and I went in and found a few students in the booths confirming this was a college town that closes the student cafeteria on Sunday evenings. I ordered a double hamburger and fries and a bottomless Pepsi Cola. That hamburger tasted better than filet mignon.

I didn't know anyone in the room and no one seemed overly anxious to meet the geek. Then, Martha Collingwood walked in, ran over and gave me a big hug and cheery welcome and slid into my booth. She had heard I was coming and had seen Jack on the campus earlier. Seeing her was like having my guardian angel walk through the door to rescue me. She said she wanted to show me the campus and introduce me to anyone who might be around. And that she did. I began to feel right at home.

When I got back to my room, around 9 pm, I went straight to bed. Around 11 pm, I woke up when the door opened and a huge guy came in, took off his clothes and crawled into bed with me. "What's going on? Is this one of those polio hallucinations," I wondered? Just as I was about to get up in protest, this guy said, "I'm your roommate, and I just got back from football practice."

This was an unexpected gift. A built in friend I was unaware of. Who snored! All night! I finally fell asleep as the sun was coming up, and when I regained consciousness, I found my new "friend" had left a note telling me he was moving into a fraternity house, leaving me at home alone.

Things picked up once I hit the campus. Two fraternities seeking support for their sagging GPAs, no doubt, had heard about this smart kid from the third world of western Kansas and had sent their representatives to woo me. They worked in teams of two — both guys in each pairing were pre-med or pre-dental — knowing in advance that I was heading toward a medical career if chemistry or math didn't get in the way. Jack, on the other hand, hid out in his room in Joliffe Hall avoiding social contact that might distract him from his studies. I pledged Zeta Chi, a local fraternity founded in 1905 by a group peppered with pre-ministerial students, and it had a long tradition of scholarship, including two Rhoades scholars and a Boston University professor who was a close personal friend of Laurence of Arabia. Zeta Chi was the current winner of the academic scholarship cup among fraternities. Six weeks later, I persuaded Jack to join Zeta Chi as well, and he moved into "Horn Hall" with me at the semester break.

Dr. Bill Rice welcomed me to the Chancel choir and accepted me as a private voice student as well. A large man and former wrestler, he had a bombastic tenor voice that would crack glass when he sang a high C. Unfortunately, at a stage of his life where vocal control wanes, he continued to break glass even on double pianissimo passages. On our first meeting, he took me under his "wing" and served as an impassioned teacher, confidant and friend for the rest of my Baker experience.

Chemistry at Baker separated the goats from the bulls. Professor E. J. Cragoe, the Chairman and only member of the Chemistry Department, was tall, stiff and mean. His son, a distinguished research scientist at Merck, Sharp and Dohme, once shared with me that the family's German shepherd, a menace to their neighborhood, whimpered when his father would swat him out of his favorite chair in their home. The only time Professor Cragoe seemed to smile was when he entered the room with a pop quiz in his hands. He had taught the course for four decades and the fraternities had massive files of old pop quizzes students could study in anticipation of his surprise gifts. One problem with those quizzes was that he changed the answers from time to time just to cause a little mischief. I managed to muddle through the first year with a B; Jack got his A with ease because he had learned how to interpret Cragoe's baffling lectures. It is surprising how many future Professors of

Chemistry and industry leaders survived Chemistry at Baker. I guess it was good basic training for the rough and tumble world of corporate business and academics.

On the other hand, biology was a sanguine respite from Cragoe's rants. Professor Ivan Boyd was a kind, soft-spoken man who loved botany. Though saddled with teaching all of the biology courses, his respect for his craft and students was immediately evident despite a monstrous teaching load. Exploring the flora around Baldwin City with Professor Boyd on a field trip was like discovering a new universe just a block away. Earlier in his career, he had planted a large variety of trees on the rectangular, 12 square blocks comprising the Baker campus and had spearheaded the placement of hard maples throughout Baldwin City. In the third week of October each year, Baldwin City becomes a destination for thousands who visit to witness the blazing colors celebrated during the Maple Leaf Festival. At this time of the year, Baker becomes a sort of "Brigadoon" to alumni, a tree-cloistered oasis that pops up on the Kansas prairie for those returning to relive an enchanted period of their lives.

I took "dumbbell" English from the formidable Elsie Hively, a prune-faced, smallish woman in her mid-50s with coal black hair pulled back and piled tightly in a bun, exposing the outgrowth of naturally red hair. She had a sense of humor of sorts. She was married to the piano accompanist for Lily Pons, a famous soprano, meaning he was seldom at home, and for which Professor Hively said she was grateful. "He's a bit of a snob" were her exact words. In four years I never saw the man on the Baker campus.

I had skimped a bit in English classes in high school, getting good grades I did not deserve out of sympathy more than my competence. I think I knew the difference between a noun and a verb, although upon rereading "Homer, a Poor Man's Dog" I have cause to wonder. Our first major assignment in Hively's class was to write an essay on anything we might find interesting. I chose to write about my father's never-ending attempt to grow tomatoes in his western Kansas garden in spite of drought, grasshoppers, fierce wind and hail. He did well at growing radishes, lettuce, onions and potatoes that stayed close to the ground, but tomatoes were his undoing. On his most recent try, while I was cooking in my body cast, he seemed to have gained the upper hand. The vines were tall and lush with blossoms, and the tomatoes began to set on and grow with abandon. He could already taste the beefsteak tomatoes in his mouth, slathered with salt or sugar or eaten fresh from the vine.

Only they were not the beefsteak variety. He had mistakenly picked up seed for cherry tomatoes, as he became agonizingly aware when his crop reddened when the fruit was about as big as his thumb. Today, he would have considered his crop a huge success because cherry tomatoes decorate most salads, but in 1954, few in Johnson City, Kansas, even knew cherry tomatoes existed. He was so angry, he tore out the vines and burned them. I turned in this story and waited for Professor Hively's reception. She gave the others in the class their papers with a letter grade appended, along with her corrections. As I got up to leave, wondering if she had lost my paper, she called me to her desk and asked me to sit down next to her. When everyone had left the room, she held up my paper, bathed in red pencil notations, and waved it in my face while saying, "Grantham, this has to be one of the most grammatically incorrect essays I have had to read at Baker."

That was the blow to my solar plexus, now to prepare for the knockout punch to the chin. "But you know," she continued, "I like the story and the way you set it up. I liked that very much, so I am giving you, yes, giving you, a C minus grade, along with the challenge to work hard this semester on mastering the English language. If you succeed in communicating in writing and speaking as well as you think and tell stories, you might just make something of yourself." I guess you could call that a stiff dose of tough love. It worked, and I had a B in the course at the close of the first semester.

In a liberal arts college you are required to take a certain number of courses in the arts and sciences. My attendance in choir and voice lessons helped meet the requirement, but I needed other acculturation such as art and literature. Alice Ann Calihan, a young, beautiful, soft-spoken princess of a professor, captured my heart and uncovered my latent interest in art. The course featured early Egyptian, Middle East and European art that was fun to assimilate, but it was Impressionist art, and specifically Monet, that resonated with my spirit to the greatest degree. Without a doubt, this and the other liberal arts exposures helped to add more valences to my steak, fried potatoes and football interest profile.

My social life was full due to fraternity activities, but I did not meet or even eye a woman on campus who I thought would have anything to do with me for longer than a free lunch or dinner would take. I had put my right arm splint in the closet and worked hard not to limp on my gimpy left leg, but to no avail. During the summer break, I decided I needed to look as much like the cool guys on campus — Bill Coleman, Gerry Rutherford, Russ Dave — as a gimpy-armed, stiff-necked geek could. So I got a flat top haircut, the kind that is engineered by the barber to leave a one centimeter bald patch on the top of your head with a table-top flat crown that plunges straight down to the ears on the sides and is tapered to the neck in back. I also got a new pair of glasses with more subtle rims.

My luck changed in the sophomore year when I complained to my accompanist, Helen Hubbard, who was a year older than I and already committed to an a Air Force pilot, that I did not have a date for homecoming. Helen and I had developed a strong friendship through our meetings each week for practice and lessons with Professor Rice. As it turned out, one of her sorority roommates was in a similar fix, so she said she would ask her about "possibilities" on my behalf. The next day, Helen looked me up on campus to tell me that Carol Gabbert would be expecting a call from me.

Carol sang alto in the choir, so I knew that I could approach her after practice. I had never spoken to her throughout the previous months despite both having attended choir rehearsals and performances on a regular basis. I guess I had sorted her into that group of "untouchables," pretty girls with nice figures who would be attracted to and wooed by the cool guys, not the geeks. With a little due diligence, I learned that she had had dates with nearly all of my pledge brothers and our president during the freshman year, earning a "nice girl" tag — translation: pretty, quiet and "won't fool around." Like me, she was still searching during the sophomore year for the right match.

During the next choir practice in the campus Methodist Church, I couldn't take my eyes off of her as we sat in the choir lofts on opposite sides of the chancel. Her short, blonde hair framed powder blue eyes accentuated by deep red lips, begging to be kissed. And did I say she had a cute figure to go with her gorgeous face? My heart was skipping beats as adrenaline sloshed about my body during the rehearsal as I pondered my approach to her, fearing that upon close inspection she would decide against the venture. The preceding year, she had accepted an early invitation to homecoming from one of my brothers, only to be asked as well, a few days before the event, by the coolest man on campus, our frat president Gerry Rutherford. In Gerry's defense, he did not know she was spoken for, and she accepted Gerry's invitation without telling him. This was one determined girl! She told the other guy, another in the geek class, that she had made "other plans."

I mopped up as much of the flop sweat as I could after the rehearsal and introduced myself to Carol, asking her to accompany me to homecoming. Without hesitation she accepted, creating another epinephrine surge of expectation that surely betrayed how uncool I was. We agreed on a time I would pick her up before the football game, and I told her we would be riding with a fraternity friend who dated one of her sorority sisters.

Homecoming came and went. I shed some more "geekiness," and Carol became more animated and chatty. We started meeting frequently on campus, and I walked her home to the sorority house from time to time. I had little spending money for dates, so we hung out at the primitive Baker student union in the basement of Parmenter Hall, the oldest build on campus to which Abraham Lincoln had donated $100 for its construction. We watched television in the Zeta Chi house and, after two previous trips to the steps of the Delta Delta Delta sorority house before closing hours, I worked up the nerve to kiss her good night. And she didn't resist! Wow! More adrenaline and a couple of pounds of testosterone were released to buttress my delirious, smitten state.

About a month after we met, we sat by each other for three days on a bus that carried our choir to churches and schools in eastern Kansas and western Missouri where we performed sacred and secular music. We performed as a choir, a male quartet and soloists. It was a tiring trip even for young adults, made more tiring by incessant conversation with Carol, in which I did most of the talking. When we returned to Baldwin City, I walked Carol home and on the steps of the sorority house unloaded the big question on her — "Will you wear my lavaliere?" — which meant that we would be going steady if she accepted. She hesitated for a moment, and then calmly replied, "I don't think so."

Where was that adrenalin when I really needed it? Being congenitally uncool at such moments, I stepped back, mumbled something and turned and walked back to Horn Hall to pour out my grief to Jack who was in the room studying. "Would any woman as gorgeous as Carol ever find it in her heart to love me" was a question I asked him and myself over and over. Jack wasn't much help. He was predictably matter of fact. "Why, I love you, Jared, just not in that Eros way. Relax. Maybe you can find a nice crippled girl who will like you." It wasn't difficult to understand why Jack was attracted to petroleum engineering rather than medicine.

I was so wounded that I could not face Carol on campus and made it a point to fixate my stare elsewhere during choir practice. I licked my wounds for the next few weeks before deciding to engage her in conversation. Helen had told me during a practice session that Carol wanted to explain some things to me, and that frankly, she, Helen, was disappointed that I had been turned down. So Carol and I met in the student union, and she explained that she was very tired after the choir trip and was anxious to get to her room, change clothes and shower. She went so far as to tell me she enjoyed my company and wanted us to remain friends. I thought I might have detected a bit of an opening, but this time I kept my cool and agreed that we should "keep in touch."

When Christmas break came, I went home to Johnson City as usual. I explained to my parents I had to return to campus a few days early to "work on my cat," a dissection that was part of the comparative anatomy course. The real reason I returned was to call Carol and take her out, probably to Lawrence — a real date. My luck held. She was at home on the family farm just outside of Baldwin City, where she lived with her widowed mother and two older brothers, and she agreed to go out with me. I borrowed a car from one of my frat brothers and set out for Nirvana, the dairy farm a few blocks east of Baldwin City.

I walked tentatively to the front door and was greeted warmly by Carol's mother, Lois, and her brothers Jim and Paul. Elinor, Carol's older sister, was married and lived in eastern Missouri on a farm; Carol was the youngest. Lois's husband, Chester, had died eight years earlier at the age of 49 of an acute coronary thrombosis, leaving the family with no means of support on a farm in eastern Missouri they had rented for crop shares. With the help of family, they found another farm arrangement closer to Lois's parents who lived in Grandview, Missouri, just south of Kansas City. Lois found work at Robinson's Hardware in Baldwin City. Jim, her oldest son, ran the farm and dairy, and Paul worked at a fertilizer plant in Lawrence. The Gabberts, as my family, knew the value of a nickel and had made it through some very hard times. I felt right at home in that farmhouse among people who dressed and acted just like the souls in blue collars I grew up with. I just couldn't tell for sure what was going through their minds when they got a load of me. I'll never know why I decided to wear a black-on-white, leopard-skin, striped shirt that diverted their gaze from my geometrically perfect flat top haircut and new horned-rim glasses. We chatted for a few minutes until Carol came down the stairs to rescue me. She was simply dressed in a skirt and blouse, but gorgeous nonetheless. Thankfully all eyes focused on her. Paul, a merciless tease, commented on her "wasp waist," and I think Carol thumbed her nose at him. Everyone was smiling as we set off for Lawrence. On the way, we decided to go bowling.

I highly recommend taking your new girlfriend bowling followed by pizza, for it creates an aura of conviviality that defeats the inhibitions of a new and evolving relationship. We spent most of the evening laughing at our respective inept bowling skills as time passed much too quickly. Buoyed by Carol's playfulness and warmth during the evening, I began searching for an opening to bring up for discussion my disastrous performance on the Tri-Delta porch. As we drove south on Massachusetts Street on our way back to Baldwin City, I looked over at her and said something like, "I want to apologize for my behavior on the Tri Delta porch several weeks ago. I can't imagine what I was thinking. I'm really pleased that we've found a way to remain friends."

To which she urgently replied, "Well, are you ever going to ask me again?"

POW! The hormonal surges were back and my heart was pounding in my throat. Fearing I would wreck my friend's car, I pulled over to the curb and croaked something like, "Indeed I do! I will!" or "Are you serious?"

This time she said yes.

We believe to this day that the next two-and-a-half years at Baker were enchanted. We were both strengthened by a romance that evolved into a "pinning" in our junior year, sort of a pre-engagement engagement in which the sorority woman wears her fraternity guy's pin tied to hers. An official engagement followed at Christmas a year later. After two years at Baker, Jack moved to Kansas University to complete a degree in chemical engineering and had found Jane, forming a bond as unhydrolyzable as any chemical he might have chosen to analyze. Having survived chemistry, I worked to fill the deep vacancies in my fund of knowledge about art, literature and music. Carol majored in Home Economics with a minor in Education in preparation for a teaching career after leaving Baker.

The Gabberts welcomed me cautiously at the beginning, but when they discovered I came from the same farm community background as they, things started to lighten up. I ate countless Sunday evening dinners at Carol's home, giving me the opportunity to get better acquainted with my future mother-in-law. Lois was a "tough cookie" as they say, meaning she did not cut fools much slack. She had pinched pennies all of her life and saw value in every piece of furniture, clothing or scrap of food that she possessed. I worked hard to earn her respect, knowing that she was always watching me out of the corner of an eye.

Carol relates an incident that happened during our senior year at Baker. We had joined Lois on a visit to her parents' home just south of Kansas City where I was on display for the first time. Grandma Sherbahn personified the stern Victorian woman. She wore a puffed-sleeve house-dress and block-heeled shoes that echoed through the house as she stomped across the hardwood floors. Grandpa Sherbahn sat quietly as though in a quandary. A few weeks later, Lois told Carol she had just visited her parents alone and the topic of Carol's new boyfriend came up. Mrs. Sherbahn is alleged to have snorted, "I don't know why Carol wants to marry a cripple!"

To which my new defendant, Lois, snarled back, "There's one thing for sure! His brain's not crippled!"

When Carol told me this story, I was relieved to know that I had made it through Lois' two-year quality control test.

Jack and I saw each other less often, but we remained close friends and confidants. He told me about Jane and that she was the one he had dreamed of. I congratulated him for dreaming about something other than chemical equations and molecular structures. We decided during the senior year to ask our girlfriends the big question before Christmas. We were both certain that each would accept, as their respective expectations were not subtle. Needing advice on purchasing engagement rings, we made a visit to see my cousin Peggy who now lived in North Kansas City with her husband, Ralph Swetnam. Ralph knew of a shop where diamond rings could be bought at a steep discount. Jack and I laugh about it now, but there we were at "Zeff's Discount" examining diamonds with a magnifying lens knowing nothing about the attributes of diamonds that speak to quality. We took the plunge, bought identical diamonds, one set in white gold for Carol, the other in yellow gold for Jane. We gave the rings to our fiancées on the same evening and both accepted with great excitement. We set the wedding dates for a week apart in June so that we could reciprocate as best men. I am pleased to report that neither ring has turned a finger green after more than 50 years.

I applied to one medical school, the University of Kansas, and was accepted.

Carol applied for one job, teaching Home Economics at Milburn Junior High School, and was accepted. We were good to go!

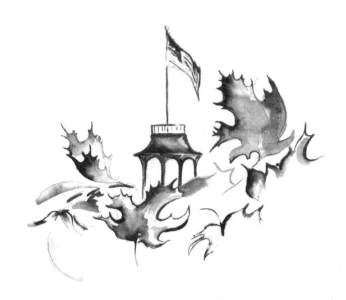

CHAPTER 13

The curiosity gene

**"Where're you walk, cool gales shall fan the glade.
Trees where you sit, shall crowd into a shade."**

On our first Sunday morning alone, as we lounged on the porch of our apartment on the University of Kansas campus atop Mount Oread, I serenaded Carol with this aria from Handel's opera "Semele" accompanied by the Memorial Campanile a few blocks to the west. After our June wedding in 1958, we spent the rest of the summer living in Johnson City so that I could work at Collingwood Grain Company and earn enough for us to get by until Carol received her first paycheck in the fall. My parents got to know Carol much better, and Annie finally had the "big sister" she had longed for to teach her about life.

This arrangement tested Carol's survival skills, as she spent most of the day at home with "mom" Ista, with occasional respites to take Annie swimming or to visit Dixie Stanton, wife of my high school chum, Leon. I came home for lunch, and that helped to break up her day and give relief from being "Istaed."

There was another reason to live at home that summer. I had developed cavities in nearly every tooth in my mouth despite brushing religiously. Virgil Ward, the family dentist located 20 miles east in Ulysses, Kansas, had recommended putting gold crowns on the teeth that were in the worst shape. He would defer payment until I had finished medical school and was in practice. So each morning, I woke up at 5:00 am and drove to Ulysses to have Dr. Ward rip the enamel off of my rotten teeth. High-speed drills were still on the inventor's drawing board, so each tooth took interminable and agonizing amounts of time to prepare. He did them in "crops" of three or four, fashioning the gold crowns in his office laboratory as he went along. Thank goodness he was an artful dentist, otherwise I might have chalked up another shaping experience.

I remember the chiseling of my upper four front teeth the best. After he cut them down to size, I resembled a hungry Dracula as he did not cover them with temporary caps. He planned to put the crowns on the following day. As had been our practice since our first night of marriage (and still is), I give Carol a good-night kiss. On this night with my exposed fangs screaming pain any time I inhaled air over them, I had rolled onto my left side with my back to her. She tapped me on my back, a signal that it was time to kiss her good night, so I turned onto my back and in the pitch black of night, she missed her target and crashed her hair rollers onto my mouth. It is conceivable that sparks jumped out of my mouth as it felt as if I had been electrocuted. I don't remember which expletives I shouted, but I do remember that Carol's only audible response was a series of stifled giggles with a muffled "I'm sorry" patched in.

My disposition and our marriage survived that summer in Johnson. At last we were free from adult supervision and alone in our first home, within earshot of the melodious and comforting sounds of the carillon wafting across the campus. Soon I was walking along Jayhawk Drive to class, following Mount Oread's glacier-chiseled crest, immersed in the resplendent beauty of the University of Kansas campus towering above the Kaw River to the north. Carol, on the other hand, was less fortunate. Each work day she had to drive 40 miles east on a narrow, hilly highway to a suburb of Kansas City where she would teach clothing to pubescent 7th, 8th and 9th grade girls in Milburn Junior High School.

On the morning of the first day of medical school, I walked the mile or so to Haworth Hall directly across from Strong Hall on Oread Drive, where the Chancellor of the University had his office. In 1958, the Chancellor was Franklin Murphy, M.D., a.k.a. *"wunderkind,"* from tony Mission Hills, Kansas, educated at the University of Kansas (AB) and the University of Pennsylvania (MD). He became the youngest Dean of Medicine in the United States upon taking the job at the perennially struggling, but proud, University of Kansas School of Medicine in Kansas City, Kansas. Since its creation, the first year of basic medical science had been taught on the university campus in Lawrence, Kansas, because the faculties in chemistry, biology, physiology and anatomy resided there. For the last three years of clinical training, students were instructed in the Bell Memorial Hospital at 39th and Rainbow Boulevard, Kansas City, Kansas.

When Murphy became Dean of the School of Medicine, he wanted to unite the basic and clinical faculties on the Kansas City campus to bring KU more in line with national trends in medical education and research. To do this, he had to convince a legislature focused on rural issues that it was in their best interest to support his vision, and so he conceived "The Kansas Rural Health Plan" with the goal of putting a physician in every town in Kansas. A key element of this package was to send each senior medical student to shadow a practicing physician for six weeks in many of the small towns throughout the state. This was sold to the politicians in the statehouse as a mechanism to give small towns an advantage in persuading these nascent physicians to practice in their communities. Coupled to the plan was a post-graduate medical education program with the slogan "Forty years not four" that took faculty from the School of Medicine on week-long trips to different communities throughout the state to deliver lectures to practitioners in their home communities.

The legislature and the governor bought into the idea and the Kansas City campus began a major expansion of the faculty and the facilities. My class would be the last to enter medical school in Lawrence. As he had done each year he was chancellor, on the opening day of class, Dr. Murphy strode across Jayhawk Drive to address the 120 new, super-charged freshman medical students. He was stunning in his double-breasted suit with his polished persona, captivating the audience with unforgettable rhetoric.

> You are about to embark upon one of the most privileged professions in history. You will literally hold the lives of your patients within your hands — an awesome responsibility. The State of Kansas wants you to remain here, to continue to learn as you practice medicine and to serve those whose taxes will have paid for most of your medical education. Our citizens need you to bind their wounds, to delivery their babies and to provide compassion to those who suffer from disease. As agents of the State of Kansas I and my staff have done our best to provide you with the most modern facilities money can buy, filled with the best teachers we can find. And at the end of this schooling, when you walk down that hill, passing by the Campanile to claim your diploma in Medicine in the stadium below, my solemn wish is that you will be just a little less dangerous than when you arrived here today.

With that he turned and walked quickly out the door across Jayhawk Drive to his office. Dr. Murphy would eventually become the Chancellor of UCLA and then the Chairman and CEO of the Times/ Mirror Corporation in Los Angeles, California. At one time, he was considered a candidate for President of the United States. He would have been a great one.

After Dr. Murphy's rousing speech, we were sorted into teams of four to fetch our cadavers. This, too, had become a ritual on the opening day of medical school. Larry Morgenstern, Bob Keys, Norman Berkley and I would spend many hours hunched over the corpse of a man in his 70s who had died of a heart attack. Anatomy is the class that takes up huge bytes of your memory simply to recall the names of muscles, nerves, blood vessels and internal organs. I once knew the names of all of the small blood vessels that contribute to the collateral circulation around the elbow. Today I find it difficult on some days to remember the name of the large vein in the bend of the elbow from which blood is usually drawn through needles for laboratory tests — the *antecubital* vein. We relied on mnemonics to make rote memory easier, at least until the quiz. The one few forget — Never Lower Tillie's Pants Mama Might Come Home — signifies Navicular, Lunate, Triangular, Pisiform, greater Multangular, lesser Multangular, Capitate, Hamate — the small bones in the hands and wrist. Why do I remember this stuff when I have never set a broken bone of any kind?

We soon settled into the routine of medical education while finding time to get acquainted with our classmates. I found the experience exhilarating and my grades proved that I was getting it. Actually, I was doing more than simply memorizing facts to be regurgitated on quizzes. I was discovering nuanced connections that were not part of the material we were supposed to learn. That made me even hungrier to know more about the functions of biologic process. I can't imagine how much more I might have learned in medical school if we had had the Internet, computers and I-Pads of today. Fumbling through the stacks of the library took precious time away from reading content.

Carol and three other wives of medical students working in Kansas City had formed a carpool. She left the apartment around 6 am weekdays and was home by 6 pm most evenings, anxious to talk about her adventuresome day. She had the strong support of an experienced principal, Dr. Jack Chalendar, who knew how to motivate and guide nervous young faculty members. Most nights, she would bring schoolwork home to grade, and I helped her as best I could. I still remember the difference between a cross-wise and a length-wise fold and how to cut on the bias. We were thrilled when she received her first paycheck, as we only had 50 cents left in our checking account. Her annual salary was $3,200 and after taxes we had about $250 a month to live on. Growing up in blue-collar families, we knew how to economize, but we still ate well. One great thing about marrying a home economics teacher is that they know how to shovel out great food within the budget.

I joined a medical fraternity for the social aspects, and this enabled Carol to get acquainted with more of my classmates' wives. We ate dinner at the fraternity house on Monday evenings. Everyone was in the same boat and needed a friendly ear to listen from time to time. There was stress too thick to cut in some of the marriages, as endless studying and small bank accounts made some of us hard to live with. Several marriages crashed that first year. Ours grew stronger.

We did have a mini-health crisis to deal with. One evening after dinner, Carol came out of the bathroom as pale as a sheet and trembling. I ran to her and asked what was going on.

"I just passed a worm!" she blurted out.

"A what?" I asked.

"A worm. It's still in the water."

Having taken parasitology at Baker, I had a pretty good idea of the kinds of worms that might inhabit the human body, so I went to the bathroom, got down on my knees and stared intently into the stool. Carol leaned over my right shoulder.

"See it! Its moving!" she gasped.

"Danged if it isn't," I replied, as I watched a whitish, string-sized object about 5-7 millimeters long move on the water from one side of the stool to the other.

"Have you been having any itching around your anus?" I asked authoritatively.

"No! Of course not," came the icy reply.

I bent down again, and the critter was still swimming in a circle from one side of the stool to the other. "Interesting," I thought, "this worm has a one-tracked mind. Maybe it's not a worm. Maybe it's just a fiber caught up in the current of a leaky toilet."

I got a long pencil and fished the "worm" out of the stool to get a close up view. It did not move on the tip of the pencil, so I put it on a piece of paper where I could poke around on it. It had a tough consistency, not compressible like a worm would be. It had to be a vegetable fiber or something like that. Then it occurred to me.

"Carol, didn't we have coconut cream pie earlier this week?" I asked.

"Yes, we ate the last of it two days ago," she replied.

"Well that undigested coconut is your worm. False alarm."

With that pronouncement, I got a big hug and a kiss. And I gained a little credibility at home as a diagnostician.

Before I knew it, I was deep into the second semester of the first year of medical school, and Carol was having a successful first year in teaching. We would soon be moving to Kansas City for my second year and needed a place to live, and I needed a job for the summer. Several of my classmates had secured laboratory research positions with basic and clinician scientists on the campus of the University of Kansas Medical School. Although Doctor Fields had stimulated my curiosity about biologic phenomena, I had never thought much about research. Rather, I was fixated on replacing the martyred physician in Johnson as my hometown had been without any medical coverage since my hero died.

In March, I visited the medical center campus to look into this "research" business as a means of earning a little extra money during the summer to supplement Carol's income. On this fateful day, I wandered, without a plan of attack, down a seemingly endless number of hallways knocking on laboratory doors in the Wahl Hall and Hixson buildings, introducing myself to everyone wearing a white lab coat that might pass as a senior researcher. After two hours, I had not turned up any possibilities — the upperclassmen attending classes on the campus had locked up almost everything before I got there. I was getting desperate when I literally bumped into Dr. George Curran who was standing in the hallway just outside of his Hixson lab. A substantial man, he stood a head taller than me, had a "strong," clean-shaven face and wore a white coat with a stethoscope in one of the pockets. He fulfilled my vision of the elegant, sophisticated physician-scientist that walked the halls of research-intensive institutions. And when he spoke to me and responded attentively and kindly to my query regarding summer employment, I felt a surge of optimism, until he patiently explained that he had already exceeded his quota of summer students.

"But you know, I think Dr. Schloerb, just down the hall that way might have something for you. Go give him a call and good luck."

"Nice man," I thought to myself while thanking him. I headed towards the next lab. I didn't hear the doctor's name that I had been told to check in with clearly, so when I got to the next lab in which another white-coated, distinguished-appearing man was standing with his back to me, I stuck my head into the open door and asked, "Are you Dr. Slur?"

He stood, clipboard in one hand and stopwatch in the other, staring intently at a fluid-filled vertical cylinder at least 5 feet long immersed in a transparent water-bath. Without turning his eyes away from the contraption in front of him he replied "Schloerb, that's S-C-H-L-O-E-R-B. I'll be with you in a minute."

Obviously, his name had been scrambled by ignorant Kansans many times before, and he calmly corrected me without breaking his gaze or moving anything else. He was about my height, slender build with a bearing that signaled sophistication. I stood frozen, fearful that I would ruin his day's work or worse. Finally, he clicked the stopwatch with a flourish, wrote the time on his clipboard and turned to me and asked, "What can I do for you?"

I introduced myself and explained that I was interested in trying my hand in research. He motioned for me to step across the hall with him to his office, where I sat in a chair in front of his desk directly across from where he was seated. He explained that he was a surgeon and was working with the new artificial kidney to treat patients whose kidneys suddenly shut down. He was also trying to perfect surgical procedures to preserve kidneys to be used for transplants and to find other treatments that would supplement failed kidneys. I don't remember any details of my contribution to the conversation, but I must not have scared him off since he promised that he would try to find something for me. He asked me to call him back in a couple of weeks.

That same afternoon, I leased a two-and-a-half room, second floor apartment on Genesse Street within easy walking distance of the medical center.

Two weeks to the hour after I had left Dr. Schloerb's office, I called him.

"What was your name again?" he asked, sounding like he'd had no idea who I was.

"I'm a freshman student who was in your office two weeks ago asking about a summer lab position. You asked me to call you back in two weeks," I explained.

"Oh, yes. Now I remember. Well it's taking longer to get anything set up for you than I had expected. You'll have to call me back in two more weeks," he said.

So I set my alarm and called again in two weeks, with the same result. Now I was getting suspicious. Maybe he didn't really want me to come but didn't have the heart to tell me. Shows you how little I knew at the time about the disposition of surgeons. For them there is no room for equivocation.

"It's me again, Dr. Schloerb. Just checking in to see if that summer position had materialized," I said on my third attempt, fearing what I was about to hear.

"Good news, Jared."

"My God, he called me by my first name. He really remembers," I thought to myself.

"You're all set. Be here as soon as you can after classes end. You'll be working with Dr. Wu Tu to get started. See you in June. Goodbye."

That was it? No other planning or long list of "to do's" before I arrive, dumb as a stump about the medical research business? I was to learn shortly about the differences in personalities between physicians and surgeons. Surgeons are always in a rush to get somewhere else. They are men and women of action whose competence is measured by how fast they incise and sew, or how many tumors they have excised and how massive they were. Physicians, on the other hand, contemplate the circumstances and have been known to stand in deep thought with their entourage by the bedside of a sick patient until a medical student or house officer either faints or dies. Speed is not important to the good physician, but getting the correct diagnosis is.

The next day, I went to the library and looked up as many of Dr. Schloerb's published articles I could find. One was especially interesting. He had determined how much water there was in a living human by infusing a stable isotope, deuterium oxide (D_2O) or "heavy water," into a volunteer's arm vein (usually a medical student or house officer). He waited a couple of hours for the fake water to distribute throughout the body and then determined how dilute the tracer had become simply by taking a sample of blood plasma. I learned from this manuscript what that long cylinder was in his office, the one he was fixated on when I first met him. Heavy water contains an isotope, deuterium, which contributes two heavy hydrogen atoms to ordinary water (H_2O). Because D_2O is heavier than ordinary water, fluids containing the isotope will sink in specialized solvents faster than ordinary water. By simply determining how fast a drop of plasma laden with D2O falls in the special solvent, Dr. Schloerb was able to calculate the concentration of the tracer in the plasma, and from that its volume of distribution, which was equal to total body water. Prior to this novel study, the only way to determine the total body water content of a human body was to weigh it, then dry it in an oven and re-weigh the residue. Medical students and house officers tended to shy away from volunteering for those experiments.

After reading more about Schloerb's work, it finally dawned on me that water makes human life possible. Without it we are dust. Since the kidneys regulate the total amount of water in the body as well as the composition of the body fluids, they are highly important as well. My affection for water had begun.

The time for Carol and me to leave our enchanted apartment on Oread Drive was soon upon us. We had survived the first year of medical school. What we did not realize was that our future preparation for a career in medicine was about to become less straight-forward than we had envisioned the day I enrolled.

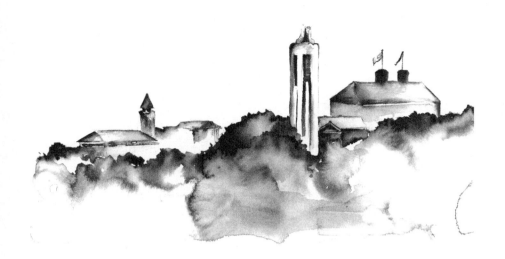

CHAPTER 14

The seduction of Jared Grantham

I arrived at Dr. Schloerb's office as scheduled to find another student sitting across his desk from him. He invited me to join the conversation then introduced me to Barbara Lukert, a senior who was beginning her research career on the same day. Barbara was from Sabetha, Kansas, a tiny village similar to Johnson City. Dr. Schloerb explained that our projects were the same in some ways. I was going to determine how to remove magnesium from the blood of dogs with the new artificial kidney, and Barbara was going to use a surgical innovation that Dr. Schloerb had devised to remove toxic wastes from the blood of patients with severe kidney failure.

When the kidneys fail to function adequately, toxic chemicals, generated by our own bodies and normally eliminated in the urine, build up in the blood causing patients to become desperately ill and die. When kidneys are suddenly starved of blood and shut down, as occurred to thousands of crushed victims of the London "blitz," death may occur within a few days. This type of rapid decline in renal function is called *acute renal failure*. More commonly, a slowly progressive renal disease like nephritis or polycystic kidney disease (Ronnie's disease) will cause the buildup of toxic chemicals in the blood over many years. Patients with insidious progression of kidney injury may not notice the toxic changes until their red blood counts decline, fatigue and shortness of breath limit their activities or they develop "fuzzy-headedness." They are said to have *chronic renal failure*.

The original artificial kidney, developed during World War II to treat patients with acute injuries, required that two hollow plastic tubes be threaded separately into an artery and a vein each time a treatment was done. After five or six treatments, all of the accessible blood vessels in the arms and legs would generally be used up. If the kidneys hadn't healed by then, the patient would die. It was not until 1970 that special plastic tubes, called shunts, were invented. These could be sewn into adjacent arteries and veins and connected outside the body, permitting repeated access to the circulation and opening hemodialysis treatment to thousands of patients with chronic renal disorders.

The artificial kidney pumps a patient's blood through a hollow cellophane tube (think sausage skin) that is bathed in a large volume of artificial plasma. The cellophane has special properties that allow tiny molecules to pass through it while leaving larger blood components, e.g. red and white blood cells, inside the hollow tube. In chronic renal failure, toxic molecules progressively build up to levels that make patients feel un-well. The toxic molecules are removed from the patient's blood as it passes through the hollow cellophane tube by a process called *diffusion*; the toxins diffuse out of the blood through the cellophane into the artificial plasma, which is then discarded. The overall process for transferring the toxic molecules through specialized cellophane membranes and into a throwaway solution is called *dialysis*;

when it involves blood it is called *hemodialysis.*

In patients with chronic kidney failure, Dr. Schloerb was using the principle of dialysis in a novel way. Instead of employing a cellophane membrane for dialysis, he used the patient's own intestine. If this invention worked, the toxic molecules in blood capillaries nourishing the intestine would dialyze into the fluid, perfusing the intestinal loop, and patients would be able to carry their "new kidney" around with them 24/7. Ironically, the first patient who volunteered for this experimental treatment had polycystic kidney disease. When I heard Dr. Schloerb mention this, I started paying closer attention.

When our meeting with Dr. Schloerb ended, he took me to his other lab in the basement of Wahl Hall to meet Dr. Wu Tu. Dr. Tu grew up in mainland China during World War II and moved to Formosa before immigrating to the United States to complete a residency in Internal Medicine. Dr. Schloerb asked me to shadow him and help out anyway I could until I was ready to take on my own project. Dr. Tu spoke excellent English but was a man of few words. He told me that he was using the new artificial kidney to study the metabolism of the mineral potassium. When the kidneys fail and potassium is ingested in the diet, it has no place to go if it cannot be eliminated in the urine. Consequently, in patients with severe renal disease, potassium levels can rise high enough in the blood to paralyze the heart unless the mineral is removed by dialysis.

Dr. Tu also used the artificial kidney to treat patients whose kidneys had failed acutely, usually from severe body trauma or a variety of toxins either ingested or mistakenly administered by intravenous infusion. Application of dialysis technology to patients was new, and important questions about how fast potassium could be removed from the body had not been addressed. Dr. Tu was attempting to answer some of those questions using the largest animal available at the time. The blood of an anesthetized mongrel dog was circulated through an artificial kidney machine just like the one used on patients in the hospital. When asked what I was doing during the summer, I enjoyed shocking the questioner by telling him or her that I used KU's new artificial kidney in the mornings to do dialysis studies in dogs, then worked with Dr. Tu to do artificial kidney treatments on sick patients in the afternoon. About one-half would ask with disgust, "You mean you used the same machine on dogs and people at that hospital?" To which I would reply, "Well, most of the time we use the machine kept in the hospital for the patients." Of course, we had two machines designated either for laboratory research or patient care, but as a matter of fact they could have been used inter-changeably because the working part of the artificial kidney was carefully sterilized.

Dr. Schloerb asked me to set up a chemical assay for magnesium and calcium, two minerals like potassium that often go haywire when the kidneys fail to function. At that time, there was no information on how fast these substances could be processed by the artificial kidney. My project was to dialyze dogs and see how well magnesium could be removed from or added to the blood stream. In retrospect, the chemical assays I had performed in high school and college chemistry classes were sloppily done compared to what Dr. Schloerb expected.

I learned how to draw small volumes of fluid into a hollow glass tube called a *pipet* with an error less than 1 percent. This part of doing research was tedious but essential to obtaining results anyone would believe. I got the magnesium assay to work perfectly, and I had learned from Dr. Tu how to prepare an animal for dialysis. So I was ready to go. The first experiment also worked perfectly. The magnesium levels in the plasma progressively fell to lower levels as the animal was dialyzed. Then, when I added magnesium to the artificial plasma bathing the artificial kidney, the magnesium levels of the dog's plasma rose steadily.

My work that summer became consuming and a little intoxicating. I was getting to do something no one else had done before. It was an exploration, like being first to climb a mountain or canoe up an unnamed stream. Carol would come to the laboratory on some evenings and help me wash glassware. She never complained about my absences, as she was having too much fun filling our new apartment with cast-off furniture. Curt Fowler, a classmate, and his wife, Connie, had moved into the apartment directly below ours. Carol and Connie became close friends and entertained one another when Curt and I were engrossed in our studies.

I repeated the dialysis experiment several times, and by summer's end, Dr. Schloerb thought we were ready to publish the results. He told me that I should write the first draft. Doing the research was great fun and the possibility that we would tell the world about it was exhilarating. But I also feared that my draft manuscript might strike the erudite Dr. Schloerb as another "tomato plant essay." I wrote and rewrote it several times before handing it to him. I hid out in the lab until a few days later when he summoned me to his office to discuss the manuscript.

Dr. Schloerb graduated from Harvard in 1941, a school whose graduates are usually articulate and write well. To my great relief, he did not fire me on the spot. Rather, he was as complimentary as a surgeon can be. He told me that I showed promise as a writer and that he would write the next draft.

This small, but monumental academic success nearly drove me to madness. I could not wait to get my hands on real patients who had problems that had not been solved. I was intent on discovering the mechanisms of their diseases and designing the appropriate cures. But first, I had to learn how to talk to troubled human beings. Apart from learning about the chemistry and physiology of the human body, in the second year of medical school we took a course called "Physical Diagnosis." It was taught by practicing physicians from the KU campus or physicians in private practices throughout metropolitan Kansas City. We were lectured on the formalisms of taking a complete medical history and performing a detailed physical exam. We were encouraged, perhaps warned is a more accurate admonishment, to read ahead and find a friend or spouse to practice on before we met our first real patient. With the help of Dr. Tu, I figured out how to use the stethoscope, ophthalmoscope and otoscope, but I didn't have a clue about what I was hearing or seeing with those tools. Poor Carol became my frequent target of abuse. It wasn't exactly the type of togetherness she had envisioned in marriage. One evening, after many failures, I actually saw her ear drum glistening brightly. Carol has *Bella donna* pupils, the type that are widely dilated, so looking into her eyes was easy, and I could study the optic nerve and retinal blood vessels until she began to cry.

The day came for my first physical examination, and I was assigned to Dr. Max Allen, a very distinguished internist, a.k.a. the doctor's doctor. I heard he was a gentleman, although I did not observe that side of his personality until the next year. In the days before health care was widely available to the poor through Medicaid, those who could not pay were seen in the physical diagnosis clinic with the understanding that they would be attended by a student and a licensed physician. I will never forget my first patient, a gorgeous 20-something, soft-spoken woman, who complained of burning when she urinated. She was very uncomfortable and anxious to get something to ease her pain. Dr. Allen watched me introduce myself to her and begin the questioning then, thinking it was probably safe to leave me alone with her, left the exam room to check on two other medical students working with him in the clinic that day.

I went down the list of questions pertinent to her chief complaint and figured out in my mind's eye that she had a urinary tract infection — another sign of things to come in my career development, perhaps? Had she been my patient today, I would have prescribed a sulfa preparation, likely over the telephone or through email, and she would have relief within 24 hours. But on that day, the pitiable thing had to sit and answer my awkward, inadequately rehearsed questions until I could fill in all of the blanks on the history and physical form. She was a good sport and tolerated my ineptitude knowing that a real physician would cure her before the day ended.

Dr. Allen evidently had a sixth sense and entered the room just as I was beginning to do the physical exam. He sat in a chair a few feet from the end of the examining table and watched intently. I would love to know what he might have been thinking as he critiqued my technique. He'd dealt with rookies hundreds of times and had suffered fools like me, most of whom proved to be educable. After examining the head and neck, it is usual to examine the chest, including the breasts in women. This young woman was unusually "well endowed" in the carnal sense, and I proceeded to apply my stethoscope to her chest without removing her blouse.

Dr. Allen sprung from his chair saying "No! No! Grantham, excuse yourself and ask the nurse to come in, remove her blouse, bra and skirt and put her in a gown to cover herself. Then we'll return."

Sheepishly, I excused myself, Dr. Allen and I stepped outside and I summoned a nurse.

"She is not your wife, Grantham!" Dr. Allen scolded. "Show her some respect and always have someone, female or male join you when you examine a gowned woman." New rules I never forgot.

When we returned to the examining room, Dr. Allen sat back down, and I placed my stethoscope on her back and systematically listened in all four quadrants as she took deep breaths with her mouth open. I could hear the air entering and leaving her lungs, but nothing else stood out. I switched to the front and did the same maneuver, avoiding her breasts as best I could. Satisfied that she had normal lungs, I began the procedure to listen to her heart sounds, only in this exam it is usually necessary to elevate the left breast to find the point of maximum cardiac thrust. Sweat beads popped out on my forehead and the tip of my nose, and I feared they would drop on my patient as I leaned over to listen. I managed a quick swipe to avoid calamity and completed the part of the cardiac exam in which the patient is seated. For the rest, she needed to lie on her back with her chest exposed so that I could listen again.

I wasn't sure what I heard, but I gambled that she had a normal heart and began to move toward the abdominal exam. This move brought Dr. Allen springing from his seat once again.

"Aren't you forgetting something important in this woman?" he queried.

I knew immediately he meant the breast exam, so I timidly began to peck around on her right breast with the tips of my fingers.

"That will never do! Here, place your extended fingers flush against her breast tissue and push it against the chest wall feeling for unusual lumps or masses. Take a systematic approach to examine all four quadrants of each breast and extend the exam into the axilla [armpit]."

He put his hand on top of mine and guided me through the exam. By the time I completed the ordeal, her breasts were no more titillating than the soles of my feet.

The rest of the exam was uneventful, as I felt for organs in her abdomen, felt the pulses in her extremities and plodded through a neurological exam as she squirmed in discomfort from bladder spasms. Dr. Allen checked her carefully, explained that she had acute cystitis possibly related to sexual intercourse and wrote her a prescription for Gantrisin, explaining that she needed to drink about 3 quarts of fluid a day and refrain from sexual intercourse for at least a week. I was surprised, when on the way out of the examining room, she paused and thanked me for taking an interest in her case, a comment that did not go unnoticed by Dr. Allen. I have often wondered if she ever came back to the KU Medical Center for any health care needs after making an uncomfortable contribution to the education of a clueless medical student.

Classes in the second year of medical school were built upon the basic science infrastructure of the first year. We studied the pathology of human diseases, the pharmacology of drugs and the microbiology of infective organisms as well as physical diagnosis. Every day we learned dozens of new medical terms and phrases as our memory capacities approached acute overload and began to short-circuit. I had been fortunate to have what some might describe as a "photographic memory" for written words and figures, but the sheer weight of new material was on occasion too much for my circuits to handle. We were forced to use corner-cutting methods to master those piles of information that we did not expect to ever use after the tests were taken. Why "Tillie's pants" survived I can't explain.

We were busy with our studies most of the time, but I had a little free time when I would sneak down to Dr. Schloerb's lab for a chat. I continued to do research during the summers, as I was excused by the Dean from certain courses that chewed up large chunks of time. In our largest study, spread over three years and done when I had time available, we determined the effects on total body mineral and water content of pronounced vomiting. Our goal was to design the most appropriate treatment for this relatively common disorder. We developed a model in dogs that mimicked the effect of an obstructing duodenal ulcer (upper intestine) in an adult or a congenital duodenal obstruction in a newborn. This work eventually led to the publication of four papers between 1963 and 1965 dealing with different aspects of metabolic alkalosis, including treatment.

Our friendship with Curt and Connie Fowler flourished, in spite of noisily padding around above them day and night. We lived relatively simple lives. Both couples had grown up in small towns and found enjoyment watching television together while eating popcorn in worn out, over-stuffed couches and chairs. For high adventure, we might drive to the bluff overlooking the Missouri River directly south where endless strings of four-engine TWA Conair airplanes targeted the short runway of Municipal Airport. During our time at the KU Medical Center, jet-powered aircraft commenced flying into Kansas City, adding to the allure of plane watching. Through the Med-Wives organization, Carol and Connie had made friends with many other women who were all in the same boat. This group got together frequently for economical evenings out.

Our first important purchase was a 24-inch window fan that saved us from suffocating in the humid 100+ degree August heat of Kansas City summers, as we had no air conditioning in our apartment. We put the fan in the north window of our bedroom so it would pull a gale from the south window directly across our bed. Our second, and somewhat frivolous, purchase was intended to establish our credit worthiness for larger needs down the road. We bought, on monthly payments, a $40 AM/FM radio with two built-in speakers, allegedly programmed to broadcast stereophonic sound. With the two speakers, about 3 inches in diameter, mounted directly next to one another, it didn't occur to us that we would have to be no larger than a mouse to get the full effect of stereophonic sound from that thing. Naive to a fault, we couldn't wait to get Curt and Connie to come to our apartment to hear the glorious sound of our new radio. They acted impressed, but I wonder if they might have realized that they were living beneath two nincompoops.

In the third year, medical students rotated onto different clinical services where they examined hospitalized patients. I was excited to begin on Dr. Allen's ward in Internal Medicine because working with him in physical diagnosis for a year gave me insight into what he expected of students. I was also fortunate that Dr. George Curran, the gentleman who had directed me to Dr. Schloerb's office a year earlier, was paired with Dr. Allen on the Medicine 2 service. The Medicine 1 service was led by an iconic physician, Dr. Mahlon Delp, who scared the bejeezus out of most medical students. Dr. Robert Manning was the "good cop" paired with Dr. Delp, a.k.a. the "brown frown." "MD, MD," as he was called by students out of his earshot, seldom smiled and was constantly upset by the ineptitude of students and house staff assigned to his service. When pressing home a failure to know whether or not a patient had urinated or passed feces in the last 24 hours, he would repeatedly pound the tip of the middle finger of his right hand on the hapless student's breastbone. No one had ever witnessed a student's death at the hands of MD, MD, but it was humiliating to be hammered in front of one's peers. Dr. Delp's harshness sent a clear message that fools would not be tolerated.

Late one afternoon, I learned that my first inpatient had been admitted to the Medicine 2 service. The resident and the intern had interviewed and examined her. Now it was my turn to spring into action and discover the pathologies they had overlooked. I introduced myself to a 60ish-year-old farmer's wife from central Kansas, a cookie cutter product of the over-worked, under-appreciated wife-factory that thrived on the high plains. I seated myself in a chair directly before where she was sitting on the side of the bed. She did not seem to be exasperated by all of the medical staff who had been around to see her; rather, she smiled and welcomed me as though she was anxious to talk to this ignoramus.

"What brings you to see Dr. Allen?" I asked.

Without hesitation she replied, "I have a numb nose."

"A numb nose," I stated, trying desperately to not have the sentence end on a higher pitch than it began.

Keeping my composure, I followed up as I had been taught.

"How long has your nose been numb?"

"About 20 years," she replied.

"And do you remember any events or circumstances that were associated with the development of your numb nose?" I asked.

"No. I just woke up with it," she replied.

Her chief complaint set me on the trail of some exotic neurological disorders, and in the course of the next 30 minutes, I asked her every conceivable question I could imagine. I stopped when I was satisfied that I was about to report a new disease — a disease that did not fit the criteria of anything that had ever been seen before. The next segment of the history was the review of systems, where physicians ask questions related to all of the organs including the heart, lungs, intestine, kidneys and so on. After an hour-and-a-half, I had filled two pages with positive answers to nearly all of my questions. This woman had symptoms in every organ system, most of long standing, and she sat there stoically reciting her aches and pains as a matter of fact.

I asked another student to be with me while I did the physical exam, expecting to find a treasure trove of pathology. I inspected, percussed, palpated and auscultated her body from head to foot and could find not even a wart. Either she was physically normal or I was hopelessly incompetent. I excused myself and wished her a pleasant night's rest.

The intern was still seated at the staff table when I returned to the nursing unit office, so I asked him, "Did you find much on Mrs. X's exam?"

He looked up from his chart and said, "Well her heart has an opening snap, indicating mitral valve stenosis, she has a retinal separation and her liver is 5 finger-breadths below the right costal margin."

"Are you talking about Mrs. X or someone else?" I asked, wide-eyed.

"Just kidding," came the reply, as he could see how upset I was getting. "She is a classic 'worried well' case. They come in here by the truck load. On the farm, it's the only way they can get any attention to their person. Their family docs usually load them up on sleeping pills or opioids, and when that doesn't work, they send them in to the super duper 'diagnosticians' at KU Med Center to make sure they haven't overlooked anything. You'll see a lot of functional illness on the Medicine 1 and Medicine 2 services. Don't despair. You'll see some really tough pathology as well. Allen and Curran are a great team."

And indeed they proved to be outstanding physicians and educators. Both had charismatic appeal with patients and the house staff. They knew their craft and could not be stumped by patients with complex disorders. I was thrilled on my last day on the Medicine 2 service when Dr. Curran pulled me aside and told me that he was very impressed with my performance and that he was aware of my interest in research. He and Dr. Schloerb were classmates at Harvard, and as I think back on it, I am certain they must have discussed me at one time or another. He strongly urged me to think about academic medicine as a career choice and to stop by from time to time to talk to him about it. His comments hit me like a blast from Mahler's Eight Symphony, and I had to struggle to maintain my equanimity. His affirmation was the vote of confidence I needed to broaden the range of realistic career opportunities in medicine.

For the second half of the Internal Medicine clerkship, I was transferred to the Veterans Administration Hospital in Independence, Missouri. It was there that Dr. Robert Brown took me under his wing and, knowing of my interest in fluids and electrolytes, suggested that I work up a new patient with a lung tumor that made vasopressin, the antidiuretic hormone (ADH). Vasopressin is normally made in special cells in the brain and stored in the pituitary gland, located a few centimeters directly behind the eyes. When we play outdoors on hot August days and lose body water as perspiration, the kidneys spring to action to hold onto as much water as they can. The amount of urine we excrete decreases sharply and becomes very concentrated, evinced by the dark yellow color. Vasopressin makes this happen by signaling the kidneys to conserve as much water as they can. In contrast, if we drink several glasses of water in a hurry, the blood level of vasopressin falls and the kidneys release more water and produce a large volume of urine that fades to a faint yellow color.

The tumor in this patient's lung was making a protein that either was vasopressin or had a structure close to it. Consequently, most of the water that he drank stayed within his body, causing his weight to increase and the salt level of his blood to decrease to dangerous levels, a condition called *dilutional hyponatremia*. Before the third year ended, I had collected four more cases similar to the first, and with Dr. Brown's help, I wrote a manuscript reporting that diuretic drugs that increased the urinary excretion of sodium chloride aggravated the low sodium state of these patients. Charmed by this fascinating disturbance of water metabolism and my experiences with Dr. Schloerb, I faced up to the fact that I was captivated by the mysterious, seductive kidney. The odds that I would be returning to practice family medicine in Johnson City were declining rapidly.

CHAPTER 15

Channeling Homer Smith

What is man, when you think upon him,
but a minutely set, ingenious machine for turning,
with infinite artfulness,
the red wine of Shiraz into urine.

Isak Dinesin

Once I decided that I would spend the rest of my life thinking about urine, I dove headlong into a self-study of the kidney. The prescient book, "From Fish to Philosopher," written by a revered renal physiologist at New York University named Homer W. Smith, became my new Bible. Homer is not a name commonly given to men, yet I have encountered it frequently. How did I come to name the dog in my first novel Homer? Was it Homer Smith using his unfathomable intellect and otherworldly powers calling me into his renal lair at an early age? Did he plant Ronnie Wilkerson behind my home in Johnson to nurture an interest in kidneys? Was Donnie Richard caught up in this scheme because of his father's first name? Did Smith's trip to Kansas University in 1943 to deliver lectures around which his famous book would be structured foreordain a vulnerable Kansan to think about urine years later?

Smith was born in Denver, Colorado, but grew up in a gritty mining town, Cripple Creek, 9,000 feet above sea level on the western slope of the Pikes Peak massif west of Colorado Springs. Records indicate that he showed an early interest in chemistry and science in general, but if you were to visit his hometown, you would wonder how a science career could be cultivated in a community of wind-swept saloons, brothels and lost fortunes on a barren landscape. Somehow he blossomed in that environment, eventually taking degrees at the University of Denver and later Johns Hopkins, developing along the way a deep interest and profound insight into the role that the kidneys played in the evolution of terrestrial mammals.

Homer Smith brilliantly envisioned the incremental stages in renal evolution forced on the kidneys by radical geological changes in the environment. Life began in the sea, evolving into animals that depend on the replication of DNA to carry the species forward. Mistakes (mutations) in DNA reproduction can confer an advantage on the organism, making it easier to adapt to an environmental change, such as living in fresh rather than seawater. In the generation of the mammalian kidney, this undirected but advantaged remodeling probably happened millions of times.

In sea animals, destined to live in fresh water and then on land, adaptation became possible when a blood filter evolved called the *glomerulus*. Ocean fish eventually found their way up fresh water streams requiring that the glomeruli excrete the large volumes of water that were ingested. Since fresh water contains vanishingly low amounts of sodium chloride and other minerals, these explorations upstream required new means to not only increase the production of glomerular filtrate but to reclaim the sodium chloride and minerals from that filtrate. Here the renal tubules connected to the glomeruli were modified to aggressively reabsorb the sodium and chloride that was being pushed down the tubule by the glomerular filters. Further down the tubule, the reabsorption of water was sharply curtailed, but not that of salt, creating the *diluting segment*, which characterizes the kidneys of all animals destined to spend most of their time in either fresh water or on dry land.

With the emergence of four extremities built on central cores of calcified bone rather than fins, locomotion was enhanced making it possible to move onto dry land for short periods. These amphibians (frogs) were constrained to live in ponds or in moist soil because their skin and kidneys had developed mechanisms to get rid of water but not conserve it. Reptiles (snakes) and birds evolved skin coverings that reduced water loss, making it possible for them to live on land as long as they had access to water. Mammals, including small rodents, man and elephants retained most of the renal features of the amphibians and the fishes and added to them a unique mechanism to limit the renal loss of water. The downstream diluting segment that appeared in frogs and fresh water fish emptied into collecting ducts that delivered the urine into a relatively large space called the renal pelvis. In mammals, the diluting segment was lengthened and curved back on itself to form a loop with a segment descending from the glomerulus called the *proximal tubule*. Together they are called the *loop of Henle* (Figure 1). The ascending diluting segment connected with the distal tubule, and in turn the collecting tubule, several of which converged to form a large collecting duct that empties into the renal pelvis. Blood capillaries also descended and ascended in a loop parallel with the tubules. This countercurrent arrangement of blood vessels and tubules allowed the kidney to set up a longitudinal *osmotic gradient,* in which the concentration of sodium chloride bathing the collecting ducts gradually increased from the tip of the papilla to the cortex. Consequently, as urine flowed down the collecting ducts to leave the kidney, it became progressively more concentrated to levels reaching up to four times greater than blood.

Our kidneys give us the freedom to wander about terra firma without access to water for several days before thirst drives us to drink. Think about it. We owe our freedom to the astonishing kidney.

Each human kidney, about the size of a man's hand, contains approximately one million nephrons, or filtering units comprised of a glomerulus, a proximal tubule, a loop of Henle (the diluting segment), a distal tubule and a collecting duct (Figure 1). The two kidneys combined process one-fourth to one-fifth of the heart's output through glomeruli that each day filter approximately 144 liters of blood plasma into the proximal tubules (approximately one barrel of plasma or about 25 times the total blood volume!). As the urine travels through the different tubule segments, glucose and amino acids are completely reabsorbed and 99 percent of the filtered sodium, chloride, bicarbonate, magnesium, calcium and potassium are also returned to the blood. What is left is excreted into the renal pelvis, and from there it courses down the ureters to the urinary bladder where it collects until it is passed to the outside through the act of urination.

The elegant human kidney is the product of random environmental pressures that were brought to bear upon our antecedents as they evolved spanning millions of years. As evolution generated animals with more complex body plans, the kidneys adapted to regulate the composition and volume of the body fluids. Claude Bernard, the famous French biologist, was the first to write about the *milieu interieur*, i.e. the sea within. Called the extra-cellular fluid, or sea that the body cells and tissues "swim" in, its composition and volume are precisely regulated by the kidneys. Homer Smith captured the elegance of the mammalian kidney with this passage:

> The human kidney manufactures the kind of urine that it does, and it maintains the blood in the composition which that fluid has, because this kidney has a certain functional architecture; and it owes that architecture not to design or foresight or to any plan, but to the fact that the earth is an unstable sphere with a fragile crust, to the geologic revolutions that for six hundred million years have raised and lowered continents and seas, to the predaceous enemies, and heat and cold, and storms and droughts; to the unending succession of vicissitudes that have driven the mutant vertebrates from seas into fresh

water, into desiccated swamps, out upon the dry land, from one habitation to another, perpetually in search of the free and independent life, perpetually failing, for one reason or another, to find it.

Urine is in fact slightly-used blood plasma that contains the waste products of body metabolism and the minerals we have ingested that are not needed when body stores are replete. Since 99 percent of the filtered blood plasma is reabsorbed by the tubules and returned to the blood, the kidneys have a dominant role in adjusting the levels of essential minerals in the blood stream, and therefore, are necessary for the other vital organs to function properly. One would be hard-pressed to make a case for intelligent design in respect to how the human kidney came to pass. Long before Creationists claimed that a supernatural force created everything in nature, Homer Smith asked a key question:

> What engineer, wishing to regulate the composition of the internal environment of the body on which the function of every bone, gland muscle, and nerve depends, would devise a scheme that operated by throwing the whole thing out sixteen times a day — and rely on grabbing from it, as it fell to earth, only those precious elements which he wanted to keep? Only nature can be so extravagant, and only in the light of historical perspective can we understand her extravagance.

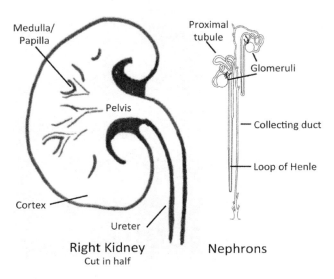

Medulla/Papilla

Proximal tubule

Glomeruli

Pelvis

Collecting duct

Loop of Henle

Cortex

Ureter

Right Kidney
Cut in half

Nephrons

Above left. Kidney. *Cortex* is outermost and *medulla/papilla* is innermost. *Pelvis* collects urine that flows to the ureter and then to the urinary bladder (not shown). Above right. *Nephrons* are the functional units, about 1,000,000 per kidney. Blood plasma filtered by *glomeruli* passes into *proximal* tubules where precious components are returned to the blood by reabsorption leaving waste products in the urine. The *loop of Henle* generates dilute urine, which flows into the *collecting ducts* where it is extensively reabsorbed when anti-diuretic hormone is present in blood. When water is drunk in excess, lowering ADH blood levels, large volumes of dilute urine are excreted.

CHAPTER 16

Ripening

During the senior year in medical school, I was forced to decide what I would be doing in the years to come. I was inspired by investigative medicine, but if I wanted to become a physician scientist who actually took care of patients, I would have to complete post-graduate clinical training to get a license. On the other hand, I could default to my original plan, take a rotating internship and in one year return to Johnson to practice medicine. Or I could leave clinical medicine and get a Ph.D. in physiology. Or I could do a post-doctoral fellowship in a kidney research laboratory while I made up my mind. Or I could enter a residency in Internal Medicine, completing the research fellowship after that. To break out of this quandary, I wrote to Dr. Louis Welt at the University of North Carolina, one of the world's most highly respected clinical investigators in the field of fluid and electrolytes, and asked if he would take me on as a renal research fellow. His reply was polite and straightforward. He cautioned me to either complete a residency in Internal Medicine or enter graduate school. He did not think I was ready for a research fellowship.

At Dr. Schloerb's urging, I wrote to Dr. Isidore Edelman, a former Schloerb collaborator at Harvard who was a faculty member at the Cardiovascular Research Institute at the University of California at San

Francisco. He quickly replied that while he would have a research fellowship position open, he no longer worked on body fluid metabolism. Because my letter to him emphasized my passion for body composition work that he now found *passé*, I interpreted his caveat to mean that he was not really interested in taking me on.

Dr. George Curran, who had counseled me a year earlier to consider academic medicine as a career, learned that I was looking for research training opportunities. He gave me enough money to travel to New York City and interview for a post-doctoral research position with a friend of his, a renal physiologist at the College of Physicians and Surgeons. I made the trip and sat for the interview but nothing clicked. Undeterred, my two KU mentors did not ease the pressure to get me committed to a high quality research experience before I defaulted to a career in family medicine.

Dr. Robert Berliner, Chief of the Laboratory of Kidney and Electrolyte Metabolism at the National Institutes of Health in Bethesda, Maryland, and one of the top kidney research centers in the world, visited the University of Kansas during my senior year and gave an impressive lecture on the renal handling of salt and water. I got close enough to shake his hand and thank him for visiting Kansas but had no time to inquire about research training in his lab. I wrote to him about a research fellowship and received a polite reply that his laboratory training positions were filled for the next two years, but that he would be interested in hearing from me again.

It seemed pretty clear that in the light of my anemic credentials, the stars of renal research were not jumping at the chance to invite me into their laboratories. So, unknown to Drs. Schloerb and Curran, I made a hurried trip to Des Moines, Iowa, to look at a rotating internship with my classmate Earl Gehrt. That trip convinced me that I was better suited to a residency in Internal Medicine. On the other hand, Earl was inspired, did his internship there and dedicated the next 45 years of his life to taking excellent care of the people living in Chanute, Kansas.

Dr. Stanley Shane was chief resident in Internal Medicine at KUMC and a grand role model in clinical medicine. He seemed to know everything about the patients he supervised in my care. He had just accepted a faculty position in Internal Medicine at the University of West Virginia in Morgantown, and he urged me to apply there for a residency position. This time, before I made a trip to West Virginia, I sought advice from Dr. Schloerb. First, I explained that I had decided to pursue Internal Medicine for the long term. To avoid alienating my chief advocate, I quickly pointed out that I liked Surgery but I didn't think I had the stamina required because polio had left me with a very weak right arm and hand and a weak left leg.

He understood and warmly approved my choice, then asked, "Where are you going to apply?"

"Well, I really like what I hear about West Virginia. And it's 'back east,'" I replied, knowing that Dr. Schloerb had high regard for the Ivy League schools.

"Jared, I must tell you that West Virginia is definitely not back east, at least not in the sense you seem to imply," he replied. "I'd rather see you stay here, get some more training under your belt, then go to a high end research center for your post-doctoral."

His advice, as usual, was straightforward and in my best interest. I applied to KU for a residency in Internal Medicine and was accepted. That issue resolved, I returned to my studies and the laboratory research projects I conducted in the evenings, weekends and holidays in Dr. Schloerb's lab.

During my senior year, Carol became pregnant and had to resign her teaching position when she began to "show" in December of 1961. We were excited about this wonderful gift that was due to arrive in April. During that winter, Professor Gerhard Giebisch from the Cornell School of Medicine visited the Department of Physiology and gave two lectures dealing with renal sodium and potassium excretion. His lucid presentation of complex methods and intimidating scientific data were spoken through a mesmerizing Viennese accent. I did grasp that he had inserted fine-tipped glass micropipettes into the invisible tubules on the outer surface of an anesthetized albino rat's kidney in order to collect samples of urine that were too small to see without a microscope. He then used novel analytic methods to determine the sodium and potassium concentrations in the samples. I listened in wonderment when he explained how this data had unlocked several mysteries regarding the excretion of important minerals in the urine. I was so captivated by his presentation that later in the evening I informed Carol that I was going to address our unborn child as Gerhard — Gerhard Grantham — for the remainder of her confinement.

I have come to believe that a current of history may have had a deciding role in developing the various incidents, challenges and chance meetings that have shaped my professional career. Unknown to me at the time, the glass micropipettes used by Dr. Giebisch were invented by Professor Marshall Barber, a microbiologist, on the campus of the University of Kansas, as reported in the "Journal of the Kansas Medical Society" in 1904. Barber invented the micropipette, and the micromanipulator to hold it, in order to test Robert Koch's hypothesis that germs cause infectious diseases. Barber selected a single anthrax bacterium from a broth culture with his pipette and injected it into an animal that went on to develop the full-blown disease, confirming Koch's findings and advancing the hypothesis to a theory. Barber's monumental invention is also used today to transfer nuclei from one cell to another and for *in vitro* fertilization. But sadly, only a few knowledgeable Kansans celebrate his association with the micropipette (http://kuhistory.com/articles/bacteriology-to-the-future). I would be reacquainted with and utilize Barber's micropipette just a few years after Giebisch's visit to Kansas.

Dr. Giebisch also mentioned in his lecture the work of Homer W. Smith, who was introduced in the preceding chapter. As with Barber, I did not know at the time that Dr. Smith had made a trip to the Kansas University campus during WWII to deliver a series of lectures on the physiology of sodium, potassium and water excretion. These lectures were later incorporated into his magnificent book, "From Fish to Philosopher." Why Smith chose to deliver these epochal lectures in a remote national *province* is lost to history, but my imagination draws a linkage between Dr. Smith and the recruitment, years later, of at least one Kansan to think and dream about urine.

Earl Sutherland grew up in Burlingame, Kansas, and received the 1971 Nobel Prize in Medicine for his discovery of cyclic adenosine monophosphate (cyclic AMP), a key intracellular messenger in the action of the hormone vasopressin. In subsequent chapters, you will learn that cyclic AMP is a central factor in the pathogenesis and treatment of polycystic kidney disease. The monumental milestones in science proffered by Barber, Smith and Sutherland in the heart of America evidently left residues in the ether that, like the ever-present wind, nudged a nascent scientist toward undressing the mysterious kidney.

Carol's first pregnancy had been uneventful except that she had more amniotic fluid than usual, causing her abdomen to become excessively large — it seems in retrospect that christening the fetus Gerhard had stimulated renal excretion *in utero*. Dr. Rosemary Schrepfer, her obstetrician, said the baby was also large. I had weighed 9 pounds 13 ounces; Carol was born in a farmhouse and allegedly weighed 11 pounds as recorded on a fish scale. Our baby was doomed from the start. The expected day of delivery came and nothing happened. I had taken the traditional course in Obstetrics and Gynecology and had delivered four babies without assistance. A little knowledge is a hazardous thing in medicine, and I decided to use the time-tested exercise and castor oil maneuver on Carol to get this birth rolling. We walked circles together around our small yard until she began to whine, then I had her drink a slug of castor oil. We got the desired effect from her intestines, but after two days, nothing had happened in her uterus, not a twinge.

I had not won her confidence, so Carol went back to the Obstetrics clinic, and Dr. Schrepfer admitted her to the hospital where she received some more castor oil. By midnight she was in labor, outing my obstetrical skills forevermore. She was in hard labor for eight hours before she was taken to the delivery room, the baby on its way. I stood on her right side holding her hand, and Dr. Schrepfer sat on a stool coaxing the visitor out of the birth canal. Suddenly, the head was out and then the remainder, revealing that Gerhard had a gender identity problem. Gerhard was a chubby, beautiful baby girl. Dr. Schrepfer began delivering the placenta, and as it emerged, a sudden gush of bright red blood swooshed out, decorating Dr. Schrepfer's gown and facemask and forming a pool on the floor. Carol's uterus was flaccid after the rapid decompression. There was nothing left inside the uterus to tamponade the bleeding surface where the placenta had been attached.

"Grab her uterus, Grantham!" Dr. Schrepfer barked at me. "I've got my hands full down here! Massage that uterus until you can feel it contract!"

I did as told and with my left hand reached through Carol's compliant abdominal wall until I could feel the uterus. The abdominal muscles offered little resistance having been stretched to such a great extent, so I was able to wrap the fingers of my left hand around the fundus of the uterus and "knead" it as you would work bread dough. I stole a look at Carol's face. She looked frightfully pale; yet, she was serenely beautiful knowing that she had just created a new being. Thankfully, a nurse of great experience had calmly told her that she had a girl.

"Squeeze harder, Grantham!" Dr. Schrepfer shouted out. "Pick up the pace! If you get tired move to the other side and use the other hand! Has the blood arrived?"

Blood? Not that Carol didn't need it, but they hadn't had time to cross-match her. Before I could say anything, Dr. Schrepfer said, "I ordered blood when I admitted her. I had a feeling we would need it."

"Wow," I thought. "This gal really knows her stuff."

"Okay, you can slow down, the bleeding has nearly stopped. Just give her uterus a squeeze now and then to keep it compact. It should do fine from this point on."

As the transfused blood ran into Carol faster than it ran out, she began to get color back into her cheeks and my heart rate dropped below 150 beats per minute. In medical school, I had witnessed severe bleeding but had found the strength to view it dispassionately. When the hemorrhaging person is someone you love, fright often trumps courage.

We took our newborn treasure, Janeane Marie, home after four days. Mom Ista came to help out and assisted Carol with calm assurance. Janeane was fussy and colicky, so having Mom's experienced hands to hold the baby and relieve Carol was most welcome. Carol's mother, Lois, could only help on weekends because of her job. Before long, we were in a new rhythm of life, dominated by our precious addition. My residency position was secure for another two or three years. Life was good, but that would be changing in July when I began my first year of medicine residency.

My first experience with having direct, personal contact and responsibility for patients was as the supervising resident in the emergency room at the Kansas University Medical Center. This was the largest hospital in the city, and the emergency room was always busy with patients traumatized in highway accidents, victims of the "knife and gun clubs of Kansas City" and those with diseases ignored for too long before professional help was sought. The "professional" help they received was delivered by newly minted physicians who were often experiencing these maladies for the first time. This would be my training venue for three weeks — 36 hours on service and 12 hours off to rest and recuperate, a schedule crafted by Lucifer.

I supervised four medical students, and we had the support of senior residents on the Internal Medicine, Surgery, Obstetrics/Gynecology and Pediatrics services, and their respective assigned faculty — if the crises were legitimate. Unlike today, no faculty members worked full time in the ER. This was the "make or break" experience for new resident physicians. Thankfully, we were also supported by a coterie of experienced trauma nurses who had seen nearly every ER challenge imaginable. I think they were largely responsible for any lives that might be saved by tenderfoot physicians. Emergency care by first responders was also primitive by today's standards. Ambulances were slow getting to the scenes of accidents and minimal treatment was rendered on the way to the ER. I am still haunted by the family of six who was wiped out in an automobile crash on one of the main highways. The ER was fully occupied when they arrived in ambulances, so I cleared out one examining room and triaged each new victim as they were brought in on gurneys, examining each person carefully. All were dead on arrival. In the commotion of tending to this family and advising students on what they should do for the patients they were seeing, the ambulance drivers informed me that they needed to leave the bodies and return to their posts. There was only one examining table in the room, so a grandfather and grandmother, their son and daughter-in-law and two grandchildren were unceremoniously laid on the floor and covered with white sheets until the dieners from the morgue could remove them.

At 3 am one morning, a nurse woke me and said that a patient from the State Mental Hospital in Osawatomie, Kansas, had found razor blades and repeatedly lacerated herself. I roused the medical students out of their slumber, and we examined the patient together. She had cuts on every extremity as well as the face, neck, chest and abdomen. The dozens of wounds were deep, and were it not for the compression bandages that had been applied in first aid, she would have exsanguinated. I guessed it would take four to six hours to clean and close the wounds, so I demonstrated my surgical technique to the students by cleaning and closing one of the larger wounds (I was an adequate surgeon, having operated on dozens of animals in Dr. Schloerb's lab), ordered enough sedation to keep her quiet for as long as needed and then set the students free to do their handiwork. She was a student's dream fulfilled. They did an outstanding job of making her whole again. As dawn broke, I awoke the plastic surgery resident on call to come and repair the wounds on her face.

In the second week of ER duty, Jack and Jane Reid came to town for an evening visit during one of my 12-hour breaks. Carol was delighted to show off our new baby, and I was anxious to visit with my old buddy whom I had not seen for three years. Unfortunately, I kept falling asleep during Jack's slow, halting discourses. I tried as kindly as I could, with Carol's help, to explain my rude behavior. They took no umbrage and bade farewell after about an hour.

Another late night arrival in the ER was memorable. A 300-pound elderly woman lived in a small hut with her husband in a village about 60 miles south of Kansas City. That evening, she began having grand mal seizures, and the husband called the local physician who arranged transfer to the Kansas University Medical Center without examining the patient. The woman had probably not bathed in several months and she was incontinent of urine and stool. During the trip to Kansas City, she lay on a plastic sheet and the mixture of stool and urine sloshed up and down and around her body as the ambulance lurched forward or slowed down. When she arrived in the ER, an egregious, foul-smelling patina that could not be quenched by aerosolized deodorant covered her unconscious body. Fortunately, she was no longer seizing, and I could examine her just enough to prove that her vital signs were stable. I also found a large growth behind her left eye that caused the globe to grotesquely protrude out of the eye-socket. Without any word from me, the nurses sprang into action, removing the woman's clothing and power washing her with a tap water jet that chased the mess down a floor drain. Next they scrubbed her with soap-laden brushes followed by more rinsing. Assured that she was stable, we admitted her pristine body to the surgery service, which earned me no credits from them. We learned later that the mass was a retro-orbital meningioma — a benign brain tumor — that was successfully removed.

I learned next that "medical Hell" at the University of Kansas had an annex, four floors above the emergency room, known officially as the Medicine One Service. The senior attending physician, Mahlon Delp ("MD, MD"), was such an imposing presence that grown men nearly twice his size and with academic credentials twice as numerous would step aside to let him and his trailing entourage pass in a crowded corridor. He had recently become the Chairman of the Department of Internal Medicine, a position he had coveted for many years.

Fellow Internal Medicine residents Joe Kyner and Barbara Lukert pointed out to me that Dr. Delp also had a nose for the business side of medical practice and took full advantage of the fact that the KU

Med Center was, at the time, the "Mayo Clinic" of Kansas and Western Missouri. He and Dr. Max Allen, the internist's internist on this campus, literally herded patients through the medical clinics and the hospital.

Delp and Allen had perfected what we residents called the "Blue Cross Special." Each senior resident on the Delp and Allen services lugged around thick stacks of elective admission cards for patients referred by private physicians from all across the mid-western part of the nation. Seven or eight patients would be admitted to each service on Sunday afternoon and remain in the hospital until Wednesday morning, or later if the patient developed a complication along the way.

The "worried well" were dosed on Sunday evening for radioactive iodine testing of thyroid function and received an admitting electro-cardiogram, chest X-ray and sundry skeletal films. On Monday morning at 6 am, the patients were awakened by a nasogastric tube being jammed up their noses followed by a timed gastric acid test with histamine stimulation administered by the junior resident or intern. Only one patient died of a heart attack at this initial stage, as I recall. If they were able, the patients were cleaned out for a rigid scope sigmoidoscopy exam administered by a resident physician. Bragging rights went to the resident with the highest number of cumulative inches plunged into unsuspecting colons without rupturing something. Then it was off to radiology for an intravenous pyelogram to visualize the kidneys (the patient had been without food or water for about 24 hours), followed by a quick visit to gynecology for a pelvic exam or urology for a prostate check. By mid-afternoon, additional consultants would line up outside the door to see the patient. When the evening tray came around, the patient was either asleep or too exhausted to want food.

The next morning, we lowered our really "big guns" on them, including oral dye for gallbladder visualization done just before the barium enema, often with air-contrast enhancement, and finally the upper gastro-intestinal exam during which they drank more barium. These dehydrated, starving patients, now loaded with barium and iodinated contrast material, usually began begging for water. Some even questioned why they were no longer making as much urine as before. Thankfully, most of these people were relatively normal to begin with or we would have had a terrible outbreak of acute renal failure on the Medical Services. As it was, we only had about a dozen cases of mysterious acute kidney injury each year and, thankfully, all of the patients enjoyed return of normal renal function. Thank heaven, for we did not have dialysis services readily available in those days. And we obviously did not have today's informed consent procedures and quality assurance mavens nagging us relentlessly.

If they survived this ordeal, each patient would be handed their chart sealed with white tape and transported to Dr. Delp's private office on the first floor of Wescoe. After a suitable wait in full view of a busy typist-secretary, the patient would be led into Dr.

Delp's dimly lit temple of Aesculapius where he would calmly review the chart and explain what was wrong and what wasn't, with suggestions for how to take care of the problems that had turned up. Most diseases of the "worried well" were treated with strong doses of self-restraint, weight loss and strict diet control under the guiding power of the physician healer. It was not called holistic or minimalist medicine in those days, but it certainly was.

The worst nightmare for the resident physician assigned to the case during the time a patient was in MD, MD's office was the dreaded phone call, with Dr. Delp on the other end of the line barking acidly, "Grantham, get down here." Most often, Dr. Delp would have turned a page in the patient's chart and found nothing on it. I had looked after a 50ish-year-old woman who had come in concerned about her uterus. She had a myriad of other complaints, which we had competently addressed, but somehow the gynecologic exam was omitted. As I faced rustication, I decided to call for help from Dr. Kermit Krantz, a gregarious Gynecologist and Obstetrician who was also a physician scientist. He is credited with being the first to demonstrate that the kidneys of pregnant mothers adaptively increase the filtration of blood beginning early in pregnancy. He also studied the intricate anatomy of the vagina, proclaiming triumphantly in his lectures on the subject that he had proven that there were no glands in the vagina. "The only *glands* you'll find in the vagina is the *glans penis*" is a quote that is still discussed by hundreds of Kansas-trained physicians who gather in Kansas City on Alumni Day to reminisce.

Within 10 minutes after Dr. Delp's call to the floor, I had the patient in Dr. Krantz's office. He examined the patient, gave me a wink, and her, a pat on the fanny, while telling her and all the office staff within ear-shot that she had one of the finest uteruses he had ever seen. She went home a happy woman, and I went to Jimmie's Jigger for a beer or two.

In what little free time I had, I played with Janeane and helped Carol with the usual tasks assigned to men, the most egregious being the diaper pail detail. Disposable diapers were unheard of, so we used cloth diapers that had to be recycled after use. They were rinsed in the bathroom stool to dislodge the larger goodies, then placed in the diaper pail until it was full or the ammonia generated by the collision between urine and poop made it difficult to breathe in that room. I would lug the pail to the washing machine in the basement and dump the contents in, add detergent and slam the lid shut trying to not add my own stomach contents to the mix. In an hour, the pristine diapers were placed in the dryer where Carol could remove them without suffering back strain or retching. In the fall, Carol informed me that number two was due to arrive the following July. Well at least I was doing something constructive in the home besides the diaper pail detail. But relatively soon I would need a bigger bucket.

In October, amidst the Med One Service onslaught, Mr. Khrushchev decided to cause some mischief by putting atomic warheads on rockets in Cuban silos that could reach all of the major cities in the continental United States. Carol and I listened to the frightening news as we held our precious Janeane in our arms, worried that we might become separated should a bomb land on or near Kansas City. The Kansas City metropolitan area was a target because atomic warheads carrying megatons of explosive power were resting in silos ringing the city. We decided that should we become separated, we would meet on the Baker University campus, our safe haven, under the steps of Parmenter Hall. Fortunately, President Kennedy, the first president for whom we voted and loved, found a sensible solution and the Cuban missiles were removed.

In the spring of 1963, I decided to reopen my search for a research fellowship position to commence after the second year of residency. I was finding Internal Medicine residency interesting, but I longed to do more than physical examinations and treating the "worried well." Solomon Papper, at the University of New Mexico, was doing interesting studies in patients with alcoholic liver disease and renal insufficiency. He also had a good, if not outstanding, reputation as a clinical investigator reflected by membership in the "right" academic societies. Carol and I paid a quick visit to Albuquerque, New Mexico, in the spring to check things out. Dr. Papper offered me a position on the spot, which I found most encouraging because it indicated that perhaps my luck had changed. I deferred my response until I could discuss it with Carol, who had been driving around the city while I was with Dr. Papper. When Carol and I reconnected after the interview, she let me know that it was fine for me to move there but that she and the children would not be coming along. She being a woman of firm convictions, I politely informed Dr. Papper that while his program was appealing, I had chosen another pathway. I did not tell him that I had not a clue where I would end up.

But others at KUMC were at work on my behalf out of view. When I told Dr. Schloerb about the encouraging letter I had received from Robert Berliner at the NIH, he and George Curran got together to discuss my situation and came to the realization that they were Harvard classmates of Jack Orloff, who had just taken over as Chief of the Laboratory and Electrolyte Metabolism at the NIH when Robert Berliner moved up to be Director of the Intramural Research Program in the National Heart Institute. They encouraged me to write to Berliner inquiring about a fellowship beginning in July 1964, and they would send separate letters of support. Within two weeks, I had a letter from Berliner telling me that he had changed positions at the lab but that Jack Orloff was very interested and would most certainly take me on. After a brief celebration with Carol, I ran to Dr. Schloerb's office to share the news with him. He telephoned Dr. Curran who appeared in the office shortly, the two conspirators struggling to control their own glee knowing they were largely responsible for helping this country bumpkin get a foot in the door at the leading kidney research laboratory in the world.

CHAPTER 17

Transition

In the spring of 1963, I attended the Federation Meetings in Chicago with Dr. Schloerb where he was to give a report of our work and where I was to meet and visit with Maurice B. Burg, M.D., a new faculty member of the Kidney and Electrolyte Laboratory at the NIH. I had been informed by Dr. Orloff that I would be working with Dr. Burg when I joined the lab the following year and that Burg and I should explore mutual interests when we met in Chicago. Translation: Dr. Burg would be determining if I wore shoes, spoke without torturing English grammar and had enough sense to know which end of a pipette to put in my mouth.

I met Dr. Burg in front of his hotel late one afternoon.

"Are you Dr. Burg?" I asked the short man wearing a sport shirt open at the neck and holding a FASEB meeting book.

"Moe Burg," he replied. "Are you Jared?"

The nickname, Moe, caught me off guard.

"Yes, indeed," I replied as we shook hands.

And following that inauspicious beginning, we set off to stroll the sidewalks of Chicago and discuss our collaboration that would last for the five years I was employed by the National Institutes of Health.

Moe graduated from Harvard College and from the Harvard School of Medicine. He completed a residency in Internal Medicine but had decided to make a career in laboratory research following a fellowship at the National Institutes of Health with Jack Orloff. He and Orloff used the unusual anatomy of the chicken kidney to demonstrate that potassium was secreted from the collecting ducts into the final urine. The studies were elegantly designed and convincing, warranting high praise from the renal physiology community. To obtain urine in a chicken, one has to place a small plastic tube in the cloaca, the chicken's rectum. The experiments were conducted early in the morning when cloacae were commonly packed with feces derived from food eaten the day before. Moe, who proved to be a brilliant researcher, had agreed to return to the NIH on the condition that he would never again have to suffer the indignity of having a chicken shit in his face at 7 am.

Moe had certainly paid his dues as mentee to the great Jack Orloff who was mentee to the great John Peters at Yale. On meeting Moe for the first time, anyone would quickly understand that he is inordinately bright and creative. I fear to imagine the kind of first impression I made on him. However, I must have passed muster, or I wouldn't be writing this narrative. When I think about it objectively, I've got to give him, Schloerb and Curran huge credit for sensing my latent capabilities more keenly than I would have judged myself. My mentors evidently saw in this physically distracting hulk, an inquisitive, intuitive and passionate person with raw intellect willing to take some risks to discover something new.

Before we concluded our meeting in Chicago, Moe explained that the mammalian kidney is anatomically complex and many of the functional units are inaccessible to direct study. He thought he had found a way to release the tiny functional units, called *nephrons*, from their confinement and was working out ways to study them individually. The small size of the nephrons — about the diameter of human hair — raised some formidable analytical challenges that he thought the technological development resources of the NIH could help us solve. His descriptions of the research objectives were lucid and the strategies to achieve them were brilliantly conceived. I left our meeting ablaze with excitement and eager for the next 15 months to vanish.

I excitedly reported to Carol the details of my meeting with Moe Burg and what a remarkable opportunity this would be for us if Moe's vision worked out. Carol was pleased to know that we would have stability built into our lives for several years and that I was excited about the challenges ahead. I kept this information to myself and pledged Schloerb and Curran to secrecy as well. Were Dr. Delp to learn of my defection from the Internal Medicine residency program before completing the third year, he would have me drawn and quartered, or more likely assigned to call every weekend and holiday during the coming year.

I girded my soul for the second three-month rotation on the "Old Man's" service. Carol was hugely pregnant with our second child, and with a toddler at home, she had her hands full. I didn't get much sympathy when I reported to her about my daily duels with MD, MD. She went into labor early one morning. I took Janeane to a friend's house for safekeeping and admitted Carol to the Obstetrics unit. Dr. Schrepfer was on vacation and the Chairman of the department, Kermit Krantz, M.D., would be her attending. Dr. Krantz was as well known on the KUMC campus as Dr. Delp. Students believed that he was bipolar, only they never got to see the hypomanic side of him. Indescribably intelligent, he commanded the conversation in every room of every size. Arrogant beyond imagination, he touted the operations he co-invented endlessly but in a way you never forgot. His lectures were replete with explicit photos and cartoons of female genitalia, and his discussion of the physical act of intercourse, from the woman's perspective, took more turns and twists than "Fifty Shades of Grey."

Frankly, I was relieved when I learned that the experienced Dr. Krantz would be delivering our next child. I left Carol and climbed two flights of stairs to join my Medicine One team. Dr. Delp would start rounds in two hours and there was much preparation ahead. On schedule, he appeared on the fourth floor like an apparition, summoning his followers to join him. We had just begun rounds when a ward clerk pulled me aside to tell me she had word from Dr. Krantz that I was needed in the delivery room.

I approached Dr. Delp cautiously and asked permission to leave rounds and join my wife who was delivering our child. I was pleased that his response was, "Oh, of course, Grantham, we can handle this."

I went to the delivery deck and stuck my head in. Carol lay in stirrups, her feet pointing away from the door. Dr. Krantz stood between her legs, his hands feeling something out of my line of sight.

"Jared, I'm so glad you are here. This is the biggest God damn baby I have seen in quite a while. He has a shoulder dystocia, and I may have to fracture his collar bone … " Just then, he stopped talking and the next thing I knew he was juggling a baby in his hands trying desperately to not drop it on the floor. He finally got control and tossed the child across Carol's lower abdomen so she could see her new son.

"Well, Jared, I made that maneuver up on the spot, but I misjudged how fast he would squirt out when the dystocia was relieved. When I saw his fat cheeks peeking out at me, I knew I was in for a struggle to bring his shoulders along. But I tried a new trick I had been thinking about for years, and it worked! Almost too well!"

I thanked him profusely and reached for Carol's hand. This time there was no blood on the doctor or on the floor and it was smooth sailing from there on out. Jared Taylor Grantham weighed in at an even 10 pounds.

During the second year of Internal Medicine residency, I supervised first-year residents and medical students. I discovered I had a knack for teaching at the bedside using techniques I borrowed from some of the older attending physicians in the department and adding a few of my own. Compared to Dr. Delp's military inspections, tours with other attending physicians were civilized walks in the gardens of disease and the worried well. In March, I was awakened at 5 am by a telephone call from a man whose voice I did not recognize.

"Is this Jared Grantham?" a strident voice barked out.

"Yes," I replied hesitantly.

"Have you rented a place to live — yet — for next year?" the questioning, unidentified voice asked briskly.

By now I had emerged from the haze of sleep and asked, "Who's calling?"

"Jack Orloff, Jared. Guess I didn't introduce myself."

"Oh, good morning Dr. Orloff," I replied.

"I'm not interested in your morning. I want to know if you have a place to live this coming July."

"No, not yet. We are just getting to that."

In a calmer tone he said, "Well I think I have something you can't refuse. I've had a change in plans and will take a sabbatical leave beginning on July 1st. Moe, with the help of Dr. Berliner, will supervise your activities while I am away — which brings me to the real reason I called. I have a house that would be perfect for you, and I'm discounting the rent to $200 a month. What do you say to that?"

My head was in a spin. I had never met this man and only knew what Moe Burg had said in passing, something like "Jack sets the tone of the lab," perhaps a warning I didn't pick up on at the time.

"Can I take some time to think about it?" I pleaded.

"Okay. Take an hour then call me back." Then he gave me his call-back number and ended the call.

Carol had listened intently to the brief conversation. We had information from NIH that I would receive an annual stipend of $8,000 a year, tax free, or $666.66 per month. (Isn't there something foreboding in the Book of Revelations about sixes?) I was currently receiving $200 per month as a resident, and we were borrowing extra money to get by. Rent in Kansas City for our small house was $80 per month. We had hoped to find a similar living arrangement in Maryland, leaving us with enough cash each month to shop away from the dented can and day-old bread sections of the supermarket. We wrestled with the high rent and the responsibility of living in the boss' house with two small, messy children, but came to the view that this "bird-in-hand" was worth the risk. It would certainly reduce the hassle of looking for a place to live while bunking in cheap motels. I called Dr. Orloff back, confirmed the rent and agreed that we would take possession of the house on July 1st.

About a week later, Carol informed me after a late dinner one weekend evening that our third child would be arriving in December. We decided to keep this one a secret until it arrived as a blessed family Christmas gift, sparing us our parents' vilification for several months.

I finally found the courage to notify Dr. Delp that I would not be completing the third year of residency. I explained that I had secured a fellowship position in the top kidney physiology laboratory in the world, and while I hated to leave Kansas, this was an opportunity I had to take. I apologized for any difficulty my absence might cause in scheduling resident assignments the following year. He did not throw me out of his office, but I could tell that he was peeved. He wished me well, and that was that.

July was soon upon us. The movers came on June 29 to take our furniture and assorted possessions. The truck was supposed to take three days to get to Rockville, Maryland, timed to deliver our furniture two days after the Orloffs moved out. We left the same day with clothing, two small children and assorted essential items crammed into our tiny Ford Falcon. I had $150 in my pocket to last us until my first fellowship check arrived in late July. We made it to Effingham, Illinois, the first day before the babies became too restless to go on. We spent a restful night in a small motel and hit the road the following day, still buoyed by the excitement of our grand venture into the great unknown. Carol had never been this far east before; I had been to New York City, Philadelphia and Washington on Boy Scout trips or to attend science meetings, but the responsibility for taking my little family into unchartered territory was beginning to hit me. Somewhere in Ohio, Taylor threw up his breakfast and lunch feedings all over Carol, and Janeane began crying in sympathy. We had to stop at a service station to clean everyone up, costing us valuable time. We had planned to spend another night on the road, but as we got closer to the major population centers just days before the 4th of July weekend, we found that all of the motels had posted no vacancy signs, so we ploughed ahead into the night. We headed south into Maryland until I began seeing double near Frederick. I pulled into a rest stop at 3 am and promptly fell asleep along with the other passengers in the car.

I was awakened at 6 am by the morning sun blazing into my face. The others stirred awake and soon the car was enlivened by the cries and screams of hungry babies. I started the car and drove to the nearest restaurant where we could clean up and fill some empty stomachs. We were a greasy looking lot; nonetheless, they let us enter the restaurant without restraint. By 10 am, we had reached the road leading to the Orloff house in North Rockville. Most of the houses were single-story, ranch-style buildings with adjacent carports, set on ½ acre lots filled with tall pine, fir, maple and oak trees. Carol and I looked at each other in wonderment at our good fortune.

A car was parked in the driveway to the Orloff house, which was unexpected as the family was supposed to have moved out. I parked our car and went to the door, unshaven, rumpled and still smelling of baby vomit. Dr. Orloff responded to my knock and stepped outside.

"Your stuff arrived yesterday, and we don't leave until tomorrow," he said as though that was the expectation.

"Dr. Orloff, we were expecting to spend the night in your house. I've got a wife and two kids who had to sleep in the car last night," I replied.

"Well, I'm sorry, but our mover got screwed up on the dates, and your stuff arrived too soon. Oh, they had to put your furniture in storage and said it would cost $150 to retrieve it after the 4th of July."

I was pretty good at crisis management, but this had turned into a colossal nightmare, and I was about to lose my equanimity when Dr. Orloff's wife, Dr. Martha Vaughan, stepped outside and brought civility to the meeting.

"I overheard what was said, Jared. You and your family must be exhausted. Let's go inside and get organized," she said as she took charge of the botched first meeting between my new boss and me.

I introduced Carol and the children to the Orloffs, and we went indoors to tour the house and to work out a few details of the verbal rental agreement. Jack and Martha both had sabbatical assignments in Paris making them unavailable should we have problems with the house. They had enlisted Dr. Bob Scow, their neighbor across the street who also worked at the NIH, to be my go-to person to help with any problems we might have with the house. Jack made it very clear to me, several times during this meeting, how much they loved their house, even wiping a doorknob with a cloth after Janeane had tried to turn it. I feared that my career in science would depend less upon my scientific prowess than the condition in which we left Jack's crystal palace.

We found an inexpensive motel where we could spend a couple of nights until the house was empty. I telephoned the moving company to set the date for returning our furniture and confirmed the storage costs. I could not convince them that the error was theirs. I also telephoned the Interstate Commerce Commission and spoke to a bureaucrat who explained that I had just experienced a common practice of moving companies that added to their bottom lines. I had no recourse, except to outsmart them as one woman did in a similar situation. When the movers arrived to deliver the stored goods, she insisted that they unload it before she would give them the check. When they returned to collect the check, she stuffed it into her bra and then defied them to get it. Unfortunately, I did not own a bra.

I had insufficient funds to pay the movers, so I called my parents who had bailed us out so many times before. They would send the money, but the holiday was a problem in getting it to us quickly. There was no Western Union outlet nearby and there was no overnight mail delivery. So they sent the check by snail mail, leaving me with only one other option. I would have to ask my new boss, Moe Burg, a man I had only met once in Chicago more than a year ago, for a short-term loan. I found him in his laboratory on the sixth floor of Building 31 on the NIH campus, shook his hand, said hello and "Could I borrow $150 dollars for a few days?"

To his great credit, he didn't blink and said, "Yes, if I have sufficient funds in my checking account." Moe was just a notch above me on the income scale at the NIH, and lacking family wealth, $150 was a sizable amount of money to have just lying around. I shall be forever grateful for the faith he showed in me with so little to guide him as to my integrity. Then I explained why I needed the money for the short term. He said he would look at his checkbook that evening. He thought he could help but just needed to confer with his wife before writing the check. I apologized profusely for ruining our first meeting in the laboratory.

On the 5th of July, I opened a checking account with a deposit of Moe's $150 check and $50 dollars of my diminishing cash. The movers came on schedule. We had made the transition, the children had beds to sleep in and we were all clean.

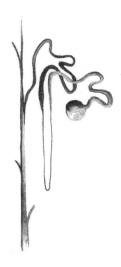

CHAPTER 18

Let the fun begin

The site selected by President Harry S. Truman to house our federal government's premier medical research programs in more than 30 buildings is just north of Bethesda and directly across the Rockville Pike from the National Naval Hospital. Building 10 had two long corridors 14 stories high intersecting at the middle. The north-south building housed patients with different types of disease referred there because scientists were doing research to learn the cause of that disease and design treatments. The laboratories were housed along the east-west corridor; the Laboratory of Kidney and Electrolyte Metabolism occupied 16 rooms on the sixth floor.

The K & E Laboratory was one of the original research groups created on the campus by James Shannon, an early Director of the National Institutes of Health. Shannon, a highly respected physician-scientist had made pace-setting discoveries in renal physiology with Homer Smith.

He recruited a rising star, Robert Berliner, M.D. of Columbia University, to be the first director of the K & E lab. Berliner recruited Jack Orloff, M.D. out of John Peters' laboratory at Yale to join him as full-time faculty. Together, they performed brilliantly-crafted studies to solve some of the more interesting secrets that until then had been locked up within the kidney; these revelations had lifted the K & E lab to the summit of renal research programs in the world.

When I arrived in the laboratory in 1964, there were still thousands of unsolved questions buried within this mysterious vital organ. Their simple kidney-bean shape camouflaged a mind-boggling tangle of functioning elements within them. As mentioned earlier, kidneys regulate the volume and the composition of the body's fluids by filtering each day about 150 quarts of blood plasma through specialized blood capillaries called *glomeruli*, no bigger than the tip of a pen. The clear filtrate flows into a network of hollow tubes each smaller than a human hair (see Figure Chapter 15). There are about a million glomeruli attached to tubules about an inch long in each kidney that are responsible for reabsorbing back into the blood all but about one quart of the filtered plasma; the left-over filtrate eventually leaves the body in the act of urination. To complicate matters, each tubule is composed of at least 12 sequential sections that do different types of work in the course of making the final urine.

What was known then about kidney function was largely based on the pioneering work in the 1940s of Homer Smith, at New York University, and Robert Pitts, at Cornell University, who studied intact, functioning organs in living animals. The kidney was treated analytically as a "black box" into which blood entered through the renal artery and came out through the renal vein, while urine mysteriously emerged into a *ureter* that drained the liquid into the urinary bladder from whence it was expelled periodically. The formation of the final urine depends, therefore, on precise coordination among several functional components to maintain the composition and volume of our body fluids relatively constant day to day.

The specific mechanisms within a kidney that contribute to the miracle of urine formation from blood were poorly understood until scientists began to look inside the "black box." Shortly before World War II, A.N. Richards, at the University of Pennsylvania, developed miniaturized Barber-type glass pipettes to sample urine from single glomeruli, tubules and blood vessels in a frog's kidney, an animal that could be easily manipulated in the laboratory. Finally in 1956, Carl Gottschalk, M.D. applied micro-sampling techniques to the kidneys of a warm blooded species, the white rat, at the University of North Carolina. The kidney was exposed through a surgical incision and the magnified surface viewed through a high-powered microscope. Specialized tools called micro-manipulators, also designed by Barber and similar to the robotic surgical techniques used today to reach poorly accessible places in the human body, were used to puncture the hair-sized tubules, withdraw urine from them and analyze the chemical content. In Germany, Karl Ullrich, M.D. was but a year behind Gottschalk when he independently developed a technique to thread tiny plastic tubes up the terminal collecting ducts of a rat kidney to sample urine within the inner kidney medulla. The lid of the "black box" had been opened, and there was a rush to set up micro-puncture and micro-catheterization laboratories in major universities in the United States and Europe, each attempting to determine how the tubules modified the urine as it passed through them.

Scientists quickly learned, however, that they could only sample tubules that reached the surface of the kidney leaving most of the deeper and highly important downstream segments hidden from view. To solve this problem, Moe Burg thought he could dig the buried tubules out of the kidney where they could be directly studied by micro-techniques — the project he had discussed with me nearly two years earlier in Chicago. He had begun to work on the method to isolate the individual tubule segments from rabbit kidneys because he had been using that for some previous work on cellular electrolyte and organic acid transport. He had been joined a year earlier by Maurice Abramow, M.D., a post-doctoral fellow from the University of Brussels. The day I walked into the lab to begin my career as a renal physiologist, I found Moe and Maurice staring into an inverted compound microscope, the kind where the objective lens is beneath the glass slide holding the target of interest. There were vertical pillars on either side of the microscope supporting a derrick-like device that held a stainless steel object resembling a large bullet. A glass tube, tapered sharply to a point, stuck out of the "bullet" into a chamber containing liquid mounted on the stage of the microscope, a rig similar to the one Marshall Barber had used at the beginning of the 20th century to corral a single bacterium from culture medium.

Moe asked me to look into the microscope and describe what I saw. After fidgeting for a long time to adjust the binocular lenses, I finally got situated. I had forgotten that everything appears backward when viewed in a compound microscope, so I was immediately scolded for saying left when I meant right. What I saw was breathtaking. There in the dish, magnified 200 times, lay a curly segment of a proximal convoluted tubule. Nearby was the tip of the micropipette that expanded to a larger glass shank that was held by the silver bullet. The micropipette tip had a second hollow glass tube inside it, and I could see clear fluid running out of it into the yellow-colored medium in which the tubule was bathed. I explained what I saw, which was substantially correct, pleasing Moe and Maurice. Moe then explained that he was going to try to advance the inner perfusion pipette into the open end of the tubule. This maneuver, at a magnified level, would be like sticking the nozzle of a hose in a gasoline filling station into the fill pipe of your car, except that everything had to be done backwards with surrogate arms and hands.

Moe struggled with this maneuver for several minutes before joyfully getting the fluid to run into the tubule. But elation suddenly changed to chagrin because the lumen of the tubule opened for just a short distance before a hole developed, causing the perfusate to leak into the bath. He showed us what was going on and then collapsed in the chair by his desk. This was the fourth gorgeous tubule he had literally blown up.

Moe explained that the perfusion device was a micropipette within a micropipette made of two concentric lengths of glass tubing. The working ends of each micropipette were shaped under microscopic vision with a micro-forge, an instrument consisting of a platinum wire connected to a current source that melted the glass allowing the operator to sculpture the tip. Assembling the pipets and filling them with solution was a challenge because microscopic pieces of lint, pollen or dandruff could plug up them up. Everything had to be carefully filtered. Needles used to fill the micropipettes and other paraphernalia had to be wiped down with lint-free paper. Each "blow up" came at the expense of at least two days' work.

My first job was to calibrate a pump that would be used to drive the fluid continuously through the tubules once we figured out how to keep the wall from leaking. Calibrating a pump held little excitement, but at least I was in the mix of technical development with colossal upside potential. And to his credit, Moe turned me loose to try any new twist I could think of to move the project along.

Moe was becoming increasingly frustrated by this "Groundhog Day" experience. Dr. Berliner checked in each afternoon to get the bad news after he had met with his team down the hall where they had discussed the results of the latest experiment. The gloom hung heavily over the Burg team, for if we could not perfuse the tubules, we would likely find ourselves staring at more chicken rectums.

Moe had cautioned Maurice and me to be cautious in what we said to Dr. Berliner about failed experiments because he would use any excuse to cut the lab budget now that he was Intramural Director of the Heart Institute. Berliner's reputation for penury was legendary. I saw him in action one afternoon when storied NIH heart surgeon A.G. Morrow, M.D. caught up with Dr. Berliner in a lab I happened to be working in. Dr. Morrow said he needed to purchase one of the new electronic calculators at a cost of several thousand dollars to compute some standard deviations from his latest clinical series of heart surgeries. Dr. Berliner asked him how many cases he had, and Morrow replied 15 and showed Berliner the list.

"You don't need a calculator to do that!" Berliner scoffed, as he took the list and manually did the calculation in a few minutes, including a t-test of statistical significance. I don't know if Dr. Morrow ever got his electronic calculator for the next set of data. Today he could purchase one for less than a dollar.

Sometimes it helps to have a farm boy on the team who will do the experiment only an ignoramus could think up. It was Moe's practice to isolate the tubules by cooking thin slices of the kidney in an enzyme that dissolves the connective tissue that holds the tubules together in the intact kidney. Moe wondered if the enzyme was dissolving an outer supporting layer around the tubule that was holding the cells together, sort of like the casing that holds sausage together. Hearing this, I decided to try a radically naïve approach and dissect the tubules without using the enzyme treatment. To soften the tissue and separate the tubules from each other, I infused liquid agar (Jello-like substance) into the renal artery of a rabbit until it started squirting through the outer surface of the kidney. With fined-tipped tweezers in each hand, I began tearing apart thin slices of rabbit kidney in a fluid-filled dish under a microscope, and to my surprise, several intact proximal tubules popped out of the gooey mess right away. I jumped up and ran into Moe's room to tell him the exciting news. He confirmed my observation and we celebrated our good fortune by setting up another pipette and showing that fluid would now run down the full length of the tubule, spilling out the other end without rupturing the wall. I was overjoyed that I had made my first substantial contribution to the project, and I assume Moe was pleased to discover that I was not a total ignoramus.

We did several more dissections, learning that we didn't need to infuse agar beforehand or use any digesting enzyme. We were ready to take this project to the next level, but we only had primitive equipment Moe and Maurice had pilfered from other labs in Building 10. With Dr. Orloff on sabbatical leave, we had to go to Dr. Berliner with requests for additional equipment and supplies. We were at a disadvantage because Dr. Berliner had a large section of the K & E lab under his watch, and he spent most of his free time talking to his fellows. John Dirks was the leader of a dog kidney micro-puncture study to determine if the proximal tubules were involved in regulating how the kidneys excrete sodium, a key question of the day. Rex Jamison, also a Berliner fellow, and his team were using micro-puncture to study renal concentrating mechanisms in the medulla of rat kidneys. Barry Brenner would join the group later in the year to use rat renal micro-puncture to study the regulation of sodium excretion. The Berliner group always had smiles on their faces because of the rewards that fell their way for experiments that generated interpretable data.

The Orloff labs were transitioning from studies in living animals to simpler models of renal tubule function. For the time being, the chickens had been put to roost and new technologies were being developed to assist in understanding the cellular mechanisms of renal salt and water transport. This kind of research is like taking an automobile engine apart piece by piece in order to understand how energy derived from gasoline is used to propel the car forward.

Joe Handler headed teams that were investigating the mechanism of action of antidiuretic hormone (ADH, also called arginine vasopressin, AVP) using the urinary bladder of a South American toad as a surrogate for the collecting duct of the mammalian kidney. When a toad hops around on dry land, its urinary bladder helps prevent desiccation by reabsorbing water from the urine back into the blood. ADH released into the blood speeds up the absorption of water from the urinary bladder before the toad can get rid of it by urination. Shortly before I arrived, Joe Handler and Jack Orloff had published a pivotal study using toad urinary bladders that strongly implicated a role for cyclic AMP in ADH-dependent water absorption. ADH, the first step in the cascade increased the levels of the "second messenger," cyclic AMP, which in the third step caused pores to open in the bladder cells allowing water to be reabsorbed back into the blood. The "steps" within the cascade of events initiated by hormones like ADH contribute to a process called signal transduction, where mediators in the extracellular fluid outside of individual cells interact with intracellular effector molecules, in this case water pores.

The ADH-mediated conservation mechanism is essential for mammals to survive during periods when access to water is limited. We see this mechanism in action most clearly when we have been playing or working outdoors in hot weather with little water to drink. The urine typically turns dark amber as the excreted chemicals responsible for the usual pale-yellow color are concentrated by the kidneys. When we drink enough to quench our thirst and reduce plasma ADH levels, our urine returns to a pale yellow hue because some of the water we drank escapes into the urine and dilutes the yellow pigment. Animals that live on dry land typically produce urine that is more concentrated that blood plasma. ADH, the hormone that regulates water reabsorption by the renal tubules, is present in the bloodstream to a variable degree, day in and day out.

The toad bladder work had revealed important new information about how ADH regulates the urine concentration mechanism. The fellows working with Joe Handler were feeling pretty chipper about their futures in American science. By contrast, Moe Burg and his team were struggling to develop a method to study renal tubules outside of the animal, and after two years, had no numbers to share with anyone. Consequently, when Dr. Berliner made his "laboratory rounds" at 3 pm each afternoon, he would stroll through the Burg lab to make sure we were all coming to work.

Moe decided it was time to show Dr. Berliner our latest success starting with gorgeous examples of proximal tubules and collecting ducts lying free in the dissection dish. The *cope de foudre* would be an elegant perfused tubule visible in the compound microscope. The 3 pm witching hour arrived and on schedule the enigmatic Dr. Berliner, referred to as "The Eagle" by his coterie, came to roost on a perch while looking into the microscope at the individual dissected tubules. Moe stood by verbally guiding Dr. Berliner's examination of several carefully arranged, twisted tubules magnified about 100 times. We couldn't tell for sure, but we think Berliner may have smiled as he studied the once invisible segments he had built hypotheses around for so many years.

Moe invited him to move to another microscope where he examined, at even higher power, the perfused proximal tubule with fluid running through it and out of the broken end. Dr. Berliner remained cool and matter-of-fact while reviewing the jewels of our stunning, breakthrough technology. A man of almost divine vision, I think he immediately grasped the effect that this hard-won advance would have on the course of renal investigation. Completely undressing the mysterious kidney might jeopardize the powerful mystique that had captivated the brightest and the best to study it. As a famous ecdysiast once said, "Take all your clothes off and he will forget you. Leave a few things on and he will think about you for hours." Renal physiologists had become leaders in academic medicine by reasoning how the kidney made urine; now they were about to find out for certain.

CHAPTER 19

A thrill a month

While I was finding my way in the K & E lab oblivious to the outside world, Carol was at home alone with two small children, awaiting the arrival of a third in a few months. We had one automobile that I drove to work each day. To make matters even more challenging for Carol, my evening arrival time was unpredictable because experiments would often run beyond the usual closing time. She will tell you that she was so busy chasing after two very active children that she didn't think too much about her isolation. And I usually got home much earlier in the evenings than during medical residency. My monthly paycheck was robust by comparison to the previous poverty wages, and she had greater flexibility when shopping for groceries. On Sundays, we attended services at North Bethesda Methodist Church where we met Bob and Nancy O'Connell, who helped acculturate us to eastern seaboard living.

We continued to make rapid progress in the lab. Dr. Berliner had authorized the purchase of a unique set of micro-pipette holders made to our specifications in the NIH technical development laboratory as well as buying new microscopes and ancillary equipment. We could perfuse tubules relatively easily but had not figured out how to collect the perfused fluid that flowed out of the open end of the tubule. We were about to concede that we would have to thread a pipette into both ends when I had another hair-brained idea. Maybe the perfused tubule would seal itself within the tip of a collecting pipette that had been tapered a short distance from the tip to slightly obstruct the flow of fluid out of the tubule lumen. The increased pressure within the tubule might push the walls more firmly against the glass pipette and prevent the leakage of liquid into or out of the collecting pipette. In the quiet of a late afternoon, I fashioned a collar of glass near the tip of a pipette with the micro-forge and with this simple device gently sucked the open end of the perfused tubule into the glass pipette until it lodged at the narrow passage causing the tubule walls to be compressed against the rigid glass containment. Indeed, this created a seal that allowed perfused fluid to gather in the collecting pipette without leakage. I then inserted thin calibrated capillaries through the open end of the glass-collecting pipette to withdraw samples of the perfused fluid flowing from the tubule.

With this innovation, we would be able to determine how fast the tubule was absorbing fluid by simply subtracting the amount collected from the amount perfused. My little "breakthrough" was greeted with considerable enthusiasm, for it meant that we could now do the experiments Moe had designed two years earlier to catalogue the functions of the individual components inside the "black box." And more important to our respective futures at the NIH, it would give Dr. Berliner some more hardcore numerical data to examine.

We soon discovered that chemicals secreted by proximal tubules accumulated to extraordinarily high levels in fluid flowing through isolated segments of proximal convoluted and straight tubules, providing evidence that "naked nephrons" retained their *in situ* functions. Moe decided that he and Maurice would study the proximal tubules, the earliest segments beyond the glomerulus at the head of the nephron; I would start working on the collecting ducts, the segments farther downstream currently mimicked by the toad's urinary bladder. I remember having the strangest feeling that providence was pulling me along a certain path. With so many different tubule segments left unexplored, why did I end up being assigned the last section through which urine passes before leaving the kidney?

Christmas was fast approaching, and Carol's abdomen had resumed its audacious, fecund dimensions. I'll never understand how she managed to remain upright carrying such a load in front. She had found a woman in the District of Columbia who promised to come and stay with our children when the due date arrived. Three days before Christmas, Carol went into labor, and after what seemed like eternity, the lady arrived and Carol and I headed for Suburban Hospital near the NIH campus. In this hospital, my presence in the labor and delivery room was prohibited, so near midnight I settled into a comfy chair in the waiting room. Given the length of Carol's previous labors, I expected to take a long snooze. But at 1 am, I was awakened by a nurse pushing Carol and our new son, James Aaron, by my chair on a gurney. Carol saw me and got the nurse to pause so that I could see the little guy. Carol explained that she got into the labor room just as he "dropped out," before the doctor could apply an anesthetic. The obstetrician joined us and filled in the details of a relatively uneventful birth. I thanked him profusely, for in those days professional courtesy was extended to physicians and their families. It is ironic that James Aaron's wife, Sheila, who he would not meet for another 18 years, was born in a nearby hospital nearby five months later; however, she was not a "freebie."

I got to break the news to our parents, the one uncomfortable job I could spare Carol in this new venture. I took the expected thrashing for not telling them about her pregnancy, moving quickly to assure them that Carol and Aaron, Janeane and Taylor were doing just fine. On Christmas Day, I bundled up Janeane and Taylor for our trip to the hospital to pick up their mother and new brother, delaying our departure from home until I could rush back into the house and distribute the gifts from Santa Claus. Carol was glad to see her children, and I was glad to get our family's irreplaceable member home again. Soon we had re-established semi-controlled pandemonium in the Grantham home.

A few days later, I got a phone call from Jack Reid. He was in Washington on business and wanted to drop by and see us for a couple of days. He could not have picked a better time to come, as we were very lonesome for family and friends; moreover, this time I could guarantee that I would remain fully conscious while he was around.

Some ecstatic images will remain imbedded in my memory for the rest of my life — my gorgeous future bride as she sat directly across the chancel from me in the Baker University choir; the adorable little faces of our newborn children; and, the first time I saw a freshly-dissected, perfused, living collecting duct magnified 200 times — all love at first sight!

Renal collecting tubules have a unique and powerful role in the regulation of body fluid composition and volume, for they are the last segments through which urine passes before entering the pelvis and, eventually, the urinary bladder. They are the key elements of an elaborate renal system that conserves water so that we don't have to live in ponds, rivers or oceans. We owe our freedom to renal collecting ducts.

Moe helped by dissecting the collecting ducts while I set up the perfusion device. I positioned the tubule lengthwise in the chamber above the microscope, and fluid was infused into one end with a micropipette; at the other end, the effluent was collected in a second pipette. With the lumen inside the tubule expanded, I could adjust the focal plane of the microscope so that I could visually slice my way from one wall of the tubule to the other. I could examine the micro-anatomy of the cells lining the tubule lumen in real time and study the demarcations between adjacent cells, called *intercellular spaces*. Like a "peeping Tom," I usually stared and bonded with my naked seductress for more than an hour before attempting to do an experiment. This was a view as exhilarating as Hillary's when he reached the crest of Mount Everest. I was the first to behold the elegant anatomic beauty of a living collecting duct at such close range.

The planned experiment brought even greater rewards, for I had sat so long just ogling the collecting duct that any anti-diuretic hormone that might have been dragged along when the tubule was torn from its natural home had washed away in the external bathing medium. What I had not noticed, because it happened slowly, was that as the hormone was being removed, the cellular layer around the lumen had flattened out, making the cells less distinct than when I began the study. I had perfused a dilute salt solution into the tubule; if the wall was permeable (leaky) to water, fluid would flow in bulk across the cellular layer from the lumen into the outer bath, just like in the toad's urinary blabber. After taking several sequential samples of fluid gathering within the collecting pipette, I added antidiuretic hormone to the bathing fluid. Within five minutes, the cells lining the tubule became more distinct as they swelled and bulged into the lumen. The lateral spaces between the cells widened, indicating that increased amounts of water were flowing between the cells from the lumen into the bath. Few would fail to notice the beauty of a mountain stream as the aerated water dances around the boulders on its way to the sea, so imagine the fantastic thrill of becoming the first person in the world to see water quietly winding its way through the walls of a mammalian collecting duct under the influence of anti-diuretic hormone.

I finally broke out of my stupor and started taking fluid samples from the collecting end of the tubule. Indeed, the measurements confirmed that the tubule was absorbing more than one-half of the water perfused into it after it had been treated with antidiuretic hormone. By opening the "black box" just a little, we had proved that the principal hormone regulating water balance in terrestrial animals increases the reabsorption of water in the *collecting ducts*, case closed!

I reported the findings to the other members of the laboratory and received a polite, if not exuberant response. They, of course, had not been there to view the complete, esthetic panorama as I had and were satisfied just to see the hard numbers proving that the anti-diuretic hormone had strikingly increased the permeability of the mammalian collecting duct to water. There was undoubtedly some unspoken resentment in the "toad bladder" camp, as this new technology rendered obsolete the use of a surrogate model of collecting ducts to study cellular mechanisms of action. Were toad bladder stocks listed on the New York Stock Exchange, this would have been a good time to sell short.

This breath-taking experiment marked the date when I fell even more madly in love with the kidney and its major product, urine. She had been a seductive, mysterious and unknowable siren to so many suitors before us, and now we could undress her and discover her deepest secrets. However, so true to form in science, when I opened the lid to the "black box" and solved one of the great secrets of the long occult-collecting duct, I was greeted by another set of "smaller black boxes" that were increasingly more difficult to open.

Moe and Maurice were making progress at warp speed in the other section of the lab. They discovered that proximal convoluted tubules, the ones connected to glomeruli, absorbed fluid much faster than the downstream extensions that straighten out, the proximal straight tubules. This was an unexpected finding that "black box" reasoning and the micro-puncture of tubules on the kidney surface could not have uncovered. Bruce Tune, M.D. joined the lab and quickly demonstrated that proximal straight tubules secreted hippuric acid, an end product of metabolism, much faster than convoluted tubules, whereas proximal convoluted tubules aggressively reabsorbed glucose, explaining why this sugar is normally absent in urine. Leon Isaacson, M.D. and Sandy Helman, Ph.D. explored the electrical properties of all of the nephron and collecting duct segments we could dissect, identifying important differences between proximal tubules, ascending limbs of Henle and collecting ducts. I stayed with the collecting duct, content to understand its biology and function. The scientific ferment in Moe's expanding laboratory group made discovering important new facts about kidney function nearly a daily occurrence. Bob Berliner had even altered his afternoon flight path landing first in the Burg labs before progressing to his own.

Jack Orloff and family returned in July, and we moved our family across the street to live in the house watcher's home while he went on sabbatical. It was a convenient move for us because we had planned to train at the NIH for only two years before returning to Kansas. I had some reservations about living across the street from my boss, especially after my kid's sandy shoes had worn the finish off of the hardwood floors in the dining room.

To our relief, the family transition went smoothly, but as Moe had hinted, Jack made his presence felt in the laboratory. He was in and out of the laboratories several times a day. When he discovered that I was a closeted cigarette smoker, he would usually find his way to my lab after lunch and bum a cigarette and smoke it while railing on about politics, his son's chemistry grade or another son's proclivity to play his oboe through his nose. He told me the only reason that I got the fellowship was because George Curran had saved his life at Harvard College by tutoring him in algebra. He confessed one day that he really wanted to be a writer for the New York Times, but somehow got pushed into medicine.

Jack's wife, Martha Vaughan, is an outstanding biochemist and member of the National Academy of Sciences. She raised three boys and deserves super star status. I've often wondered if she might have advised Jack about the potential intermediacy of cyclic AMP in the action of some hormones, leading Jack to look at it in the kidney or "kidney-like" organs such as the toad's urinary bladder.

With Orloff, Berliner and Joseph Hoffman — another senior K & E lab member who worked on sodium and potassium transport in red blood cells — in attendance, the lunchroom took on a distinctive flavor at high noon. The room was about 10 feet wide with enough space for a single long table and about 20 chairs. Faculty and fellows would amble in around noon with brown bag lunches in hand. We struggled to keep Jack's hands out of our bags. One of the fellows was usually assigned to present an article from the recent renal literature and was expected to have intimate knowledge of why the experiment was done, what they found and what was wrong with it. I thought for a while that Berliner, Orloff and Hoffman were the only ones on the planet who knew how to design a controlled experiment and how to analyze it. In spite of hours of preparation, very bright fellows, including Juha Kokko with a Ph.D. in quantum mechanics, were usually stomped into the floor before the second set of data was discussed. Water boarding was a day at the beach compared to these drownings.

We quickly learned through intimidation and embarrassment the elements of perfect experimental design and execution to test a hypothesis. Once we got the hang of the game and outgrew our collective intimidation, these meetings became great fun. Each fellow sought to one-up the others with esoteric reports out of the range of knowledge of the senior faculty members. By the time a fellow was ready to leave the lab, usually after two years, he was prepared to stand before the unfriendliest academic tribunal imaginable with equanimity and grace under fire.

Dr. Berliner had made it a point to stop by my lab in the afternoons usually on his way to visit his research team. Looking back, it is clear that I had been adopted in Jack's absence. His question of the day was always, "What's new?" whereupon I would show him Polaroid photographs of beautiful collecting ducts or exciting new data from my most recent experiment. I think that early on he had sensed that we were going to succeed in our isolated tubule work, had supported it financially and now had the joy of watching the inscrutable "black box," only his intelligence could once "see" into, being opened a little bit day by day. Victims, of whom Dr. Berliner could be counted as one, learn that romancing the mysterious, seductive nephron leads to eternal bondage — a thirst for new knowledge that is never slaked, for it bears the intellectual piquancy of urine.

We worked most of the kinks out of the experimental procedure, so Moe turned over the dissection as well as the perfusion parts of the experiment to me. After setting up the perfusion system, I would spend about 30 minutes hunched over a dissecting microscope teasing collecting ducts out of a rabbit's kidney. When I had one that was satisfactory, I would transfer it to the larger, inverted microscope and attach the two ends to appropriate micropipettes. My neck frequently reminded me that it could only tilt forward at the junctions between the first and second cervical vertebrae and the 7th cervical and 1st thoracic vertebrae. Vertebrae two through seven were fused; thus, two joints in my neck were taking the brunt of the trauma of holding my head perfectly still through a dissection. I soon learned why jewelers often complained of neck pain.

The old polio wounds also complicated delicate maneuvers I needed to do with my arms and hands to perfuse the tubules. Since I was naturally right handed, I always perfused the tubules from right to left, meaning that I had to reach my right hand to a height above my head and hold it there while I advanced the perfusion pipette into the lumen of the tubule. But polio had left me with insufficient muscle strength in my wasted right shoulder to do the task. Consequently, I devised an "arm crutch" which was simply a 2-foot length of wood 2 inches thick and 4 inches wide. By extending the crutch from the upper surface of my right thigh to my upper arm near the elbow, I could prop up my arm. With the crutch in place, I could raise and lower my arm several inches by lifting the heel of my right foot in a tiptoe maneuver. This lifted my right hand into position to do the delicate maneuvers with the apparatus that controlled the movement of the perfusion pipette. At the time, I had sufficient strength in my left arm to attach the collecting pipette to the tubule without disability assistance.

As the months rolled on, I completed several studies, the most important being the demonstration that cyclic AMP mimicked the action of anti-diuretic hormone in the collecting tubule. We were also the first to show that a new bioactive lipid, extracted in Scandinavia from prostate tissue and called *prostaglandin*, would shut down the antidiuretic hormone's action to increase water reabsorption, an experiment that the Orloff-Vaughn duo had formulated.

The potent and dependable action of antidiuretic hormone on the collecting tubule was fascinating to the point that I sometimes dreamed I was small enough to swim in the stream flowing through collecting ducts while inspecting the cracks, crevices and artifacts protruding from the cells. This had turned into a real fantastic journey. When I excitedly described my day's work to Carol in these terms, I could see the concern in her eyes that her children's father may finally have slipped over the edge.

About halfway through the second year at the NIH, I was contacted by Dr. Darrell Fanestil, who had just agreed to return to Kansas and set up the first nephrology division in the Department of Internal

Medicine. Darrell had graduated from KU four years before me and was about to complete a fellowship with Isidore Edelman at the University of California Cardiovascular Research Institute, the same person I had written to years before. Darrell wanted me to fly back to Kansas and interview in the Department of Medicine for a faculty position with him in Nephrology. Carol and I were both homesick and ready to look for something closer to Kansas City. So this was an opportunity I couldn't pass up.

I flew to Kansas, met with various faculty members, most of whom I knew well, and gave a research seminar showing off our new technology that was about to revolutionize renal physiology investigation. I was politely received until I had the final meeting with Dr. Mahlon Delp (MD, MD) who was still pissed that I had left before completing my residency. Parenthetically, it was not uncommon at the time for research-oriented faculty in elite medical schools to short-circuit some of the standard training modules in internal medicine. There were many chairs of Internal Medicine who were not board certified but were held in esteem by virtue of demonstrated excellence at the bedside and their research accomplishments. Kansas was not "elite," and Dr. Delp would have none of that. He made it clear to me that he thought I was interviewing to be Dr. Fanestil's fellow and that I would need to complete my third year of residency as well. I felt hoodwinked.

I made it clear to Dr. Delp that I had no intention of being Darrell's fellow and was under the impression from Darrell that I had been invited to look at a faculty position. I excused myself from Dr. Delp's office and caught up with Darrell to recite what had transpired. He was not a happy camper, either, as he was in the process of moving his family to Kansas and felt betrayed by his new chairman.

I limped back to Maryland wondering what we would be doing in a few months when my fellowship ended. I spoke to Moe about my situation, as we had gotten along well, and I felt comfortable sharing personal issues with him. He told me he would like for me to stay on in the lab and that he was going to talk to Orloff about it. Time went by, and I heard nothing from Moe or Jack, so I figured I would be moving on to who knows where. But good fortune intervened in the form of Dr. E. B. Brown, chairman of the Department of Physiology at Kansas University Medical Center, who was visiting the NIH campus on a study section assignment and, knowing I was there, stopped by my lab to see how I was doing. I gave him the nickel tour, showing him the pictures of collecting tubules along with a condensed explanation of what the experiments meant.

He thanked me and then told me why he really had come to see me. I guess word had filtered around KU about my disastrous visit, and he thought we should talk about a faculty position in the Department of Physiology. In fact, he made me a firm offer on the spot to begin as an Assistant Professor on July 1, 1966. I was pleased, of course, but caught off guard. I asked Dr. Brown for time to visit with my wife about the move and said that I would get back to him soon. Then who should appear but Dr. Berliner, who had been a guest of Dr. Brown's during his visit to Kansas two years previously. After hand shaking and back slapping, Berliner asked Brown what he was doing at the NIH.

Dr. Brown replied, "Well Bob, I'm trying to take this young man off of your hands," or something like that. Then he explained what we had been talking about. After some more banter, Berliner excused himself and went down the hall towards his lab. I reaffirmed to Dr. Brown that I would get back to him about his generous offer, and he was comfortable with that.

About 30 minutes after Dr. Brown had left, Moe burst through the door of my lab and asked, "How does a GS 14 position here sound to you?"

In Kansas I would have "bear-hugged" him on the spot, but I defaulted instead to firmly shaking his hand.

❖

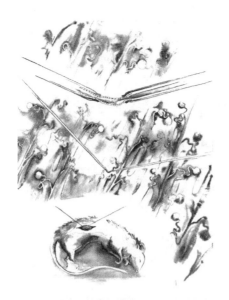

CHAPTER 20

New horizons

My salary nearly doubled in July, and we bought a second car, a Ford Falcon station wagon to accommodate our expanding family. This was Carol's car to use whenever she wanted, a degree of freedom she had not enjoyed for two years. We moved to a house in Garrett Park Estates owned by an FBI agent. It was a "cracker box" with three tiny bedrooms, a living room-dining room combo and kitchen just wide enough to turn around in comfortably. A full, unfinished basement was used for the laundry and playroom for the children. I put a 9 by 12 foot linoleum piece against a wall then enclosed the space with thin bamboo curtains to give a modicum of privacy to anyone who might sleep on the fold-out divan. For the first time in our married life, we had financial security and a job that I really couldn't call a job — it was a research paradise.

The first hint of trouble in paradise came when I explained to Moe that I wanted to pursue some morphological studies of the collecting tubules with Charles Ganote, M.D., a cell biologist I had met at a seminar. Charles was skilled at using the electron microscope, and together we dreamed up a study to explore the cellular basis of the changes I saw in the collecting ducts as they absorbed relatively large volumes of water after they were treated with antidiuretic hormone. I was perplexed when Moe told me that he was not excited about this venture.

There was an unspoken laboratory dynamic that I was slow to catch on to, a seniority pecking order beginning with Berliner, then Orloff, then Burg/Handler, ending with the new hires, Grantham and Barry Brenner. Berliner and Orloff relished their international acclaim as kings of the hill in the field of renal physiology. Burg and Handler served loyally as knights working feverishly at the bench, waiting their turns, while Barry Brenner and I were thankful just to be pawns. Beneath the overt spirit of lab camaraderie lay old wounds and jealousies ready to pop out at the most unexpected times. I learned to tread lightly among the big elephants.

The project that held Moe's highest interest was to determine if the collecting duct actively secreted potassium, an essential nutrient readily available in the diet. The kidneys are critical for regulating the amount of potassium circulating in the blood. If potassium levels rise too high, the heart will stop beating. Or if blood potassium levels get too low, patients develop severe muscle cramps and weakness and can even stop breathing. The kidneys continuously adjust the blood levels of this mineral within precise limits. Burg and Orloff had produced evidence in chicken kidneys that the control of potassium excretion rested in the collecting system, and Gerhard Giebisch had deduced as much in his micropuncture experiments. Now it was time to hone in on the cellular mechanisms by which the collecting ducts excreted potassium. This was going to be a difficult project because in addition to measuring the net movement of potassium in collecting ducts, I had to measure the transtubule electrical potential. This study would take the next two years to complete.

Jack began to loosen up around me, especially when we shared a smoke in my lab. He advised me to "soft-pedal" the electron microscope study with Ganote, a safe suggestion, because at the end of my usual experiments I usually flushed the spent renal tubule down the drain. Now, I would capture it and place it in a fixative that Charles had given me. At the end of the day, Charles would drop by my lab and pick up the specimen. The rest was in his hands. Periodically, Charles and I would meet in the NIH library, and I would examine the contraband — illegal electron micrographs of naked nephrons — that were simply gorgeous.

It didn't take long before we had enough material to warrant publication in a high-end cell biology journal. We decided to write a draft with our names as authors and give it to Jack, who would discuss it with Moe. Since Charles had done most of the legwork to develop the method for processing these tiny bits of renal tissue, we agreed that he would be the first author. We handed the draft to Jack, which he slathered in red ink before giving it back to us subversives. He had transformed our "wart" of confusing syntax and muddy grammar into a beautiful rose, which Charles and I agreed should be given to Moe. Charles passed the draft on to Harold Moses, his lab chief, who insisted that his name be included if Jack Orloff remained a co-author. This story has a happy ending, for the manuscript was published, with minor editing, in the highly-respected "Journal of Cell Biology." A year later we published a second, more analytic study in the same journal showing how water actually flows through the cellular layer of collecting ducts in response to treatment with antidiuretic hormone.

I had spent most of my time working on the potassium secretion project that Moe was interested in, but now that the detour into water had ended, I dug into electrolyte transport with renewed vigor. We eat about 50 to 100 milliequivalents (2 to 4 grams) of potassium daily primarily in meat, fruits and vegetables. The human kidney can normally excrete 10 times this amount unless there is renal disease or severe dehydration. With sudden cessation of renal excretion, as may occur after a heart attack, septic shock or serious trauma causing massive hemorrhage, the failure to excrete potassium in the urine can lead to its accumulation in the blood to life-threatening levels. Physicians have great respect for potassium among the electrolytes in blood plasma (sodium, chloride, calcium, magnesium), for it is the one most likely to kill a patient if left unchecked. Add to the fearful allure of potassium the curious fact that more than 9 grams are filtered by the glomeruli each day and promptly reabsorbed by the proximal tubules and loops of Henle. More unintelligent design! Would an intelligent engineer wastefully expend energy to pump body waste out of a river only to pump it back in further downstream?

It was believed at the time that the regulation of potassium excretion must occur somewhere between the distal convoluted tubules and the tip of papillary collecting ducts. Consequently, the collecting ducts take on enormous importance when one considers that they are the last tubule segments that can remove potassium from the body fluids.

Indeed, the isolated tubule experiments showed us that the collecting ducts could elevate the tubule fluid potassium concentration more than 10 times greater and lower the concentration of sodium to levels less than one-tenth as high as that in the fluid perfusing them. We had found the locus of the exotic *sodium-potassium exchange* process that Berliner and Orloff had postulated based on "black box" experiments in chickens and dogs. In addition to performing the tedious experiments, it took several weeks of writing and re-writing a manuscript that was published in the "Journal of Clinical Investigation."

During the year our fourth child, Joel Don Grantham, was born without incident, completing our little family. Carol juggled the four children skillfully, and I helped out evenings and on weekends and holidays. The new tubule micro-perfusion method had gained international recognition, and scientists from all over the world were coming to the K & E lab for tutorials or extended training. New knowledge about kidney function was coming to the fore almost daily as different investigators found ways to study all of the renal tubule segments as well as the glomeruli and small blood vessels. In light of the successes in the laboratory, I dared to spend more time with my family. We explored the Blue Ridge Mountains as far south as the Smoky Mountains and ventured into West Virginia.

Carol and I sang in a church choir, and I joined the Montgomery County Oratorio Society where I was cast as a tenor.

At the annual meeting of the American Society of Nephrology held in Washington, D.C. in the fall of 1968, I had a conversation with Darrell Fanestil, who had tried to hire me two years previously. He was making progress in his recruitment and had persuaded Donald Tucker, M.D., an internist with biochemistry training, and Dennis Diederich, M.D., an internist also trained in biochemistry, to join him in 1969. He was still interested in my joining him and the "good news" was that Dr. Delp had announced his retirement effective July 1969. Darrell had caught me at a vulnerable time. My future at the NIH was unclear, and Carol was desperately homesick for the Midwest lifestyle. I told him I would have to confer with Carol and that I would let him know one way or the other before the ASN meeting ended. When Carol heard the news, she was ecstatic, which came as no surprise. So we did our best to have a strategic discussion about our family life and my career opportunities in Kansas, a place most scientists flew over on their way to either coast. We concluded that I should make another trip to Kansas and retest the water.

Without notifying anyone in the K & E lab, I disappeared for a few days in order to visit the University of Kansas Medical Center. I met with faculty and gave a seminar to a small group of scientists interested in the kidneys and spoke to the Dean about his expectations. This time Kansas was ready to welcome me home and came through with an offer I could not refuse. The trip back to Maryland was much more pleasant than two years earlier. Carol and I celebrated our decision and began to make serious plans for the future. I decided to wait until the New Year to tell Moe, Jack and Bob about my new job.

CHAPTER 21

Hope and change

In preparation for my coming life as a practicing physician, uncertified in internal medicine (there were no nephrology certification boards until years later) and untested as a renal clinician, I asked my friend Bill Argy, M.D., a former "toad bladder" fellow in Jack's lab, if I could join him for renal rounds on Wednesday afternoons at Georgetown University. Bill graciously outfitted me in a special white coat, reserved for my visits, and introduced me to the fellows and internal medicine residents assigned to him. George F. Schreiner, M.D., a co-founder of the American Society of Nephrology and a former Homer Smith trainee, was the Director of Nephrology. He was the ultimate academic physician — brilliant at the bedside, skilled in the performance of renal biopsies and profoundly knowledgeable. Patients came from all over the world to be in his care. He insisted that nephrologists personally examine the urine sediment (sediment is a collection of renal debris excreted in the urine that can be examined easily at high magnification under a compound microscope) and divine the origins of the formed elements. I came to view urine sediment as analogous to fingerprints at a crime scene; you can get a pretty good idea of who the upstream culprit is if specific types of sediment appear in the urine. Perhaps Dr. Schreiner's greatest achievement was convincing the U.S. Congress, with the help of his neighbor Charles Plante, that Social Security should pay for renal dialysis and transplantation.

I had been away from clinical medicine for four years, but like learning to ride a bicycle, if you grasp the fundamentals well, you never forget how to ride, or practice good medicine. I soon learned, however, that I was far behind in therapeutics. On rounds one day, a renal fellow discussed a case of urinary tract infection, and after going through the clinical features and laboratory results, he concluded by saying, "We started the patient on Cephlan."

Cephlan? I'd never heard of it. To save face, I pulled Bill Argy aside at the end of rounds and asked, "Bill, what's Cephlan?"

He laughed aloud, then said "Jared, that's short for cephalothin, a new and powerful antibiotic that covers all kinds of urinary tract organisms and is excreted by the kidney in high concentrations."

I was also introduced to Imuran, a drug to treat transplant rejection and many others that had risen to use in only four short years. Those Wednesday afternoon stealth trips to Georgetown University were an invaluable investment of time, for they assured that I would be a little less dangerous at the bedside in Kansas than otherwise.

Moe and Jack must have smelled a rat because neither of them flinched when I told them individually, shortly after New Year's Day 1969, that I would be leaving the K & E lab in July. I thanked each of them profusely for giving me the opportunity to test my mettle and to participate in one of the most exciting research adventures in nephrology, ever. I assured them that I would work hard in the remaining months to complete all of the projects and help orient any new lab members. What I did not say to Moe, but should have, is that I was privileged to have worked for five years in close quarters with the best scientist I have ever known.

I received approval from Kansas University to purchase the intricately manufactured perfusion pieces I would need to do tubule perfusion experiments. I had persuaded Jim White, who crafted the original prototype perfusion gear in the NIH fabrication shop, that this would be a good growth business for him to set up in his garage at home. He worked on my package in his free time. Kansas University was providing generous startup funds to build the new lab and hire a research technician, but I was expected to write a grant to the NIH to pick up the ongoing costs for the years to come.

The National Institutes of Health has two major research divisions: the intramural programs that are housed on the Bethesda campus and the extramural programs that are distributed throughout the Nation on university campuses and in private research institutes. The budgets of these major divisions derive from taxes paid to the Federal Government and are allocated to the intramural and extramural programs on the basis of scientific merit as judged by peer review. It is the fairest system yet devised for deciding how to use precious money for health-related research. I look back on my initial grant application, typed without benefit of modern word-processing keyboards, and marvel at how primitive it now looks. I believed I was opening new renal territories to exploration much as Lewis and Clark did when they followed the Missouri River upstream into the wild Northwest without a map. The relative scales of our respective journeys were reflected in the opening statement of my grant: "In tiny tubules, ordinarily hidden from view, the miracle of urine formation proceeds in a quiet ritual day after day." I often wonder if the reviewers of that grant might have thought that this guy had been staring through a microscope too long.

Carol and I made a hurried trip to Kansas City in May of 1969 and purchased a house on West 82nd Street in Overland Park. It seemed huge compared to the cracker box we had been living in for three years. A new elementary school was just one block away and West High School three blocks away. I would have a 20-minute drive to the KU Medical Center. Midwesterners to the core, we were coming home at last.

A week before we were to move, Joel caught his left hand in the back door of the station wagon when one of the other kids slammed the door shut, trapping his hand. Carol had to open the door to remove his hand. He had a severe laceration across the palm surface of the third finger

— in "no man's land" — a term coined by hand surgeons for a portion of the finger where damaged ligaments and tendons can be extraordinarily difficult to fix. Carol took him to the emergency room and called me to come at once. Joel was in severe pain and was letting the world know how much it hurt. The surgeon who attended him seemed indecisive and kept probing the wound causing Joel to shriek in agony. I did not like the way things were going, so I bundled Joel up and we set out for home picking up some antibiotics on the way. We tried to gather our wits that night and decided to see how he felt after a night's rest without anyone picking on his hand. The following morning the wound did not look improved; in fact, there were clear signs of infection. I called Kansas City and spoke to Don Tucker, and together we decided that I should send Joel and Carol to Kansas City post haste and let stand-out plastic surgeon Lyn Ketchum take charge.

After calling Braniff Airlines and securing two reservations, Janeane, Taylor, Aaron and I drove Carol and Joel to the downtown airport and sent them on their way to Kansas City. The four of us were on our own, with a house to pack up and get loaded on a van and a 1,000-mile trip across the nation in torrid heat in a car with no air conditioning.

Carol and Joel arrived in Kansas City and took a cab to the KU Medical Center where they were met by Don and Virginia Tucker. Virginia, a pediatric nephrologist, was perfect for the task of calming an ailing child and comforting a suffering mom. Joel was admitted to the pediatric service and was seen promptly by Dr. Ketchum who was deeply concerned about the infection that was now raging in Joel's hand. He sedated Joel, then debrided the wound and administered strong doses of antibiotics. Carol stayed with Joel in his hospital room the first night they were there and then Carol's mother, Lois, rescued her. In two days, the infection came under control and Joel was discharged to the care of his mother and grandmother.

Meanwhile, my tiny helpers were attempting to assist me with the final details of the move. Thankfully, Barbara Disiderati, a nextdoor neighbor, took them off of my hands for extended periods and kept them fed and watered. The moving van arrived later than scheduled and the last stick of furniture was not loaded until midnight on an evening in which the temperature and the humidity remained above 95. I had made pallets for my little ones in the station wagon and around 10 pm was able to persuade them to try to go to sleep. I closed the doors to the house for the last time shortly after midnight and collapsed in the front seat of the station wagon. Five years earlier we had arrived in Maryland in the early morning, hot and greasy, and were leaving as we came.

After a satisfying smoke, I cranked up the engine and we headed to the interstate.

The kids were terrific. They sensed that this was a great adventure for our family and pitched in as best they could. We did have one early incident before we got out of Maryland. Aaron raised his head to tell me he had had an accident in his pants. Thankfully, it was only water, so I hung his shorts on the side-view mirror on the driver's side so they would dry out if the humidity ever went lower than 90 percent. Aaron slept in the buff until the sun came up. I took him into the bathroom of the filling station where we stopped for gas and wiped him down with wet towels. To a nephrologist, freshly dried urine on garments is not something to fret about. We could wash them up that evening when we stopped for the night.

By late afternoon of our second day on the road, I was beginning to see two center stripes in my lane of the highway. We had reached the outskirts of Indianapolis, and I started looking for cheapie motels. I had kept the tribe at bay during the day by promising them that we would stop at a motel that had a swimming pool. We couldn't afford the swanky Hiltons or Howard Johnsons, but I did see a sign that directed us off of the interstate to an old motel with a pool. We checked into our air-conditioned rooms with two double beds that beckoned me to lie down and take a little nap. The kids would have none of that, so we put on our swimming suits and headed for the pool. It was a small pool, but the water was clean and cold. I looked for a place where we could wade in, and I could sit by and watch my children blow off some pent-up energy.

But fate was not on my side that evening. The shallowest end of the pool was 5 feet deep, meaning that I was going to have to spend the next two hours holding onto each child as they flopped around in the water because none of them could swim. Bless their hearts, they had a grand time as I fought to stay awake. I could see the headlines: "Father falls asleep in pool; three beautiful children drown."

We capped off the evening by visiting an "all you can eat" buffet restaurant next to the motel. The kids were amazed that they could eat as much of anything they wanted. I read them a message posted on a billboard at the table where we sat, indicating that gluttony was encouraged with one caveat: Any father with a child who leaves food on the plate will be thrown in jail. I pleaded with them to not overdo it on the amounts they spooned out. We were joined in the restaurant by a clientele that was distinctly blue collar, men in coveralls and women in feedsack dresses. The food was starchy and uniformly bland "filler food." The kids loved it, especially the sugary desserts. I nearly fell asleep while eating the mashed potatoes. We made it back to the room by 8 pm, and I was asleep by 8:01 and deeply unconscious until 6 am the next morning.

We made the last leg of the journey without incident and arrived at our empty new home by nightfall. Carol and Joel joined us, having scavenged sufficient blankets and pillows from Mom Gabbert, relatives and friends. Joel's finger was showing signs of healing and didn't hurt. Our furniture arrived three days later and family life began anew for the Granthams.

CHAPTER 22

Getting started

The construction of my laboratory was behind schedule, and I would not be able to start doing experiments until September, so Darrell Fanestil thought it might be wise for me to do a clinical staff rotation in August. I was eager to wield my stethoscope again, so I accepted the assignment and set out to lead a renal fellow, Dr. Larry Benson, two medicine residents and two senior medical students into the dangerous swamps of clinical nephrology. Having been a resident physician at KUMC five years earlier, I knew the system and what the troops would expect of their attending physician. Although I had been reading clinical nephrology papers furiously for the previous three months, my fund of clinical knowledge remained the weakest component in my academic toolkit. On the other hand, I had been thinking about urine almost continuously since I made the decision to become a nephrologist years before. I knew a great deal about renal physiology and fluid and electrolyte problems; moreover, when confronted with unusual problems at the bedside, I had fine-tuned a method of systematic analysis learned in the laboratory that would often trump simple empiric wisdom. Now I wanted to help the house staff and students to appreciate and learn to use the power of quantitative thinking. This approach, known in the clinical academic club as "roundsmanship," also exposed my strengths and suppressed the weaknesses.

What Fanestil did not tell me until a week into August was that he was going on vacation, and I would be the attending nephrologist for the first related, living donor and non-related kidney transplants in Kansas. None of the KUMC clinical nephrologists, urologists or vascular surgeons had ever participated in a renal transplant involving humans, so why not me since I would be on service? The technical aspects of the procedure are straightforward and something a skilled vascular surgeon or urologist trained in vascular surgery could do without breaking a sweat. On the other hand, there is a rather large problem that the attending nephrologist must deal with after the sutures are all snugged up and the patient leaves the operating room, and that problem is called *rejection*.

Our bodies are geared to reject organisms and tissues that are not recognized as self. Bacteria, for example, are attacked immediately by white blood cells that destroy the germs literally by eating and digesting them. Red blood cells that are transfused into another human will be destroyed unless the donor cells are "matched" to the recipient through the A, B, O typing system most people have heard of. The same thing can happen when a donor kidney is sewn into a recipient. If the tissues of the donor and the recipient are not matched, the white blood cells of the recipient will attach and destroy the donor organ just like white cells destroy bacteria, except with tissues like the kidney the process is called *transplant rejection*. In 1969, the matching tests for kidneys worked pretty well for closely related persons, e.g. siblings. The first kidney transplant at KUMC would be from an older to a younger sister who appeared to be "well matched" according to the blood and tissue typing. Naivety is a powerful attribute of young academic physicians flushed with the success of opening a new approach to studying kidney function. If I knew then what I know 40 years later — that transplantation is a highly complex and perilous proposition for patients and that following two years of nephrology training, physicians spend an extra year or two in high volume transplantation programs to become a certified transplant physician — I would have run away and hid when Fanestil informed me that I was to make the maiden renal transplantation voyage in the state of Kansas. In blissful ignorance, I boarded the ship and assembled the crew.

I asked Larry Benson to cram into his head, and then into mine, everything he could find in the library on renal transplantation as fast as he could. We rehearsed the role of the renal team with the residents and students, asking them to notify their spouses or partners that they might be spending nights in the hospital for an indefinite period. We met with the surgeon, Dr. Creighton Hardin, who held the KUMC indoor speed record for opening and closing on tricky renal artery stenosis (narrowing) cases, and Dr. Winston Mebust, Chief of Urology, who would sew the ureter into the urinary bladder.

We were ready when the day came to give the patient her sister's kidney. The recipient was a cute, 19-year-old woman whose kidneys were destroyed by glomerulonephritis, a disease that attacks the blood filters in the kidneys. I scrubbed for the surgery and watched as each meticulous cut and stitch was made to prepare the lower abdomen to receive the new organ. The kidney was removed from the donor and transported to the recipient's operating room where Dr. Hardin examined the donor kidney, trimmed some excess tissue away and set to sewing the blood vessels together. In less than 10 minutes, the renal artery and the vein had been connected to the recipient's vessels, and within 20 minutes, the urologist was complaining that the "damn thing is making so much urine that it's hard to see what's going on in the wound." In this case, too much urine is a good thing! The surgeons had completed their work briskly, and now it was our turn to sweat out the rejection business.

There are two types of rejection: In the early hours post-transplant, kidneys can be lost if the recipient has an antibody in her blood to the donor's tissue that escaped detection during the tissue typing procedure. *Antibody-mediated rejection* happens quickly and destroys the kidney in a few hours. Signs that this may be happening are an increase in the patient's body temperature and a sharp fall in the rate of urine output, relatively crude indicators. The more common type of rejection is called a *cellular rejection* because the recipient's white cells become sensitized to the chemical differences between the donor and the recipient and attack the kidney tissue. This causes a fever, a slowing of kidney output and swelling of the transplanted organ, usually associated with pain beneath the incision.

Our patient did just fine, waking up from the anesthesia and smiling when she saw the bag beneath her bed filling with precious, slightly blood-tinged urine. Larry Benson and I had decided to camp out in the intensive care unit that night to monitor the urine output, armed with syringes full of anti-rejection medication if rejection dared to show its face. About midnight, the urine output started to decline, and we began to sweat. We sent urine and blood samples to the lab and waited nervously for the results. Within the hour we had figured out that this expatriate kidney had found its new home to be just fine and was doing nothing more than taking a snooze. Kidneys normally slow down urine formation at night in a process called the *diurnal rhythm*. Kidneys are normally geared to make most of the urine during waking hours and slow down at night — a wise thing to do, otherwise we would never get an uninterrupted night's sleep if we had to answer "mother nature's call" several times during the night. We relaxed when we saw the numbers and dozed off and on through the night, waking up fully with the dawn just as the new kidney started making more urine, restoring our confidence in the wisdom of the kidney. As far as I know, to date, the patient has never experienced a single twinge of renal rejection.

Our second kidney transplant patient was another matter. A sturdy, 18-year-old Kansas farm lad, he received a kidney from an un-related deceased donor, did reasonably well for about four days before he was laid out with hectic fevers, sweats, pain over the transplant and a stark decrease in urine output. We agreed that he had severe rejection and added huge intravenous doses of methylprednisolone to his standard anti-rejection regimen. The steroid quieted things down but not for long. The surgeons had struggled with this kidney when they put it in and were concerned that it may have rotated and kinked a blood vessel or the ureter. They took him back to the operating room and reopened the surgical wound. They had to rearrange the "plumbing" and were forced to leave the kidney floating freely inside his abdominal cavity, rather than tucking it into a pocket in the right lower quadrant. He required more and more steroids. We even added external beam radiation in an attempt to quell the rejection. Then he developed lung problems that appeared to be a viral pneumonia, although the pulmonary specialists weren't certain. In the midst of this baptism of fire, August came to an end and I was supposed to step aside so that Dr. Dennis Diederich could lead the nephrology parade. I was embarrassed to leave my new colleague with such a monstrous problem, but he was ready for the challenge. We had known each other since residency and had a mutual respect that was as much fraternal as professional. Under his direction, the renal team finally got to the bottom of the lung problem — indeed, the patient had acquired a cytomegalovirus infection that took several more weeks to overcome. I am pleased to report that he survived his ordeal and is alive and well today. Our first patient is a grandmother.

CHAPTER 23

"Chance favors the prepared mind." *L Pasteur*

I was out of "medical" condition and in over my head most of the month of August 1969, as I struggled to keep up with the pace required to lead a frantic clinical nephrology service. Thankfully, Dr. Schloerb was still around to encourage me when my confidence wavered. I had to learn clinical nephrology on the run and establish a research laboratory while not forgetting where I lived and the names of my wife and children. The patients always got top priority during waking hours; 3 am phone calls and overnights at the hospital tested my pluck. Upon reflection, August 1969 was probably my finest month at the bedside. I met the challenges head on, solved most of the problems with the help of some terrific house staff and managed to not kill anyone as far as I know.

I hired a young man from the Middle East to assist me in the lab, but he disappeared after only two weeks to take a higher paying job in industry. That was my good fortune, for Patti Qualizza was my next hire, a recent graduate in anthropology from Kansas University who preferred to dig up old bones and teeth on the prairie, but had to settle for a job in a medical research lab to pay off some debt. She was also an artist and had the appropriate mix of patience and dexterity to dissect renal tubules from rabbit kidneys for hours on end. Together, we outfitted our laboratory on the fourth floor of Eaton building, just 20 paces from the primitive dialysis unit where desperately ill patients received treatment. It was a great location for me because I could dash into the lab at odd times during the day from the dialysis unit or my practice on the fourth floor of the adjacent Delp building.

The animal care facility, housing the rabbits used in our research, was in another building. Patti had to make frequent trips past curious hospital visitors when she brought rabbits to the lab in a rehabbed grocery cart I had modified by enclosing the wire frame in sheet metal to hide the furry creatures inside. I didn't think anything of it, having trained at the world's leading research installation where patients and white rats shared the same floors of the massive Clinical Center. The brains of hospital administrators would explode were anything like this tried today.

During September, we got everything assembled and began doing experiments. I received double good news from the NIH: My first research grant application was approved and funded for five years as well as a five-year Research Career Development Award that carried with it salary support and a commitment from Kansas University that I would have 75 percent of my time protected for research. I failed to read the fine print on the Career Development Award because before the first year had ended, it had become obvious that KU interpreted the 75 percent time for research to mean that I would only sleep four hours each night seven days a week.

As I had stared in wonderment a few years earlier at a perfused collecting duct's response to anti-diuretic hormone (ADH), I imagined that something very special was happening within the plasma membranes surrounding the lumen. Our initial experiments led us to think that the border of the collecting duct cells in direct contact with the dilute tubule fluid flowing past them was limiting the reabsorption of water in the absence of ADH, also called *vasopressin*. Vasopressin got its name from early experiments in which extracts of the posterior pituitary gland, where it is stored, were injected into living animals causing the arterial blood pressure to shoot up. Accordingly, the active stuff in pituitary extracts was named *vaso* (vasculature, vessels) *pressin* (pressure rise) in tribute to its effect to cause blood vessels to contract and cause the blood pressure to rise.

The anti-diuretic effect of vasopressin on water excretion was discovered later when pituitary extracts were found to diminish urine output. We tend to overlook the fact that man and other animals living on dry land often go many hours without drinking any fluids. The anti-diuretic hormone stored in our pituitary glands protects us from desiccation by signaling the kidneys to conserve water. Kangaroo rats living in deserts can concentrate the solutes in urine nearly 10 times greater than in plasma. Keep in mind as you read further that except for short bursts of water drinking during waking hours, humans concentrate the urine above that of plasma 24/7. In other words, elevated plasma vasopressin levels are a constant presence in our daily lives as we move about on dry land.

The NIH findings had led us to suppose that vasopressin increased the permeability to water in or near the apical plasma membrane of collecting duct cells. The prevailing hypothesis was that vasopressin caused water pores to open in the plasma membranes of collecting ducts in contact with the urine. Since vasopressin caused the tiny, smooth muscle fibers surrounding blood vessels to contract and raise blood pressure, I wondered if the hormone might also cause the sub-microscopic fibrils called *actin*, near the apex of collecting duct cells, to also contract. Opening the water pores in the plasma membrane would likely be associated with a physicochemical change that I could measure. I decided that I would try to explore this hypothesis in my first independent research project at Kansas. I chose an unorthodox method to test an unorthodox idea. I set about to measure the stiffness or deformability of the collecting duct plasma membrane in contact with the tubule fluid flowing past it in response to vasopressin.

The simplest analogy I could imagine was a collecting duct cell as large as a simple water-filled balloon. If I used a finger, or a more sophisticated tool that records force, to indent the balloon, I could record the amount of energy that would be required to deform the wall of the balloon a predetermined distance. Ophthalmologists do this simple test routinely to diagnose glaucoma. Equations have been developed to quantify the stiffness (deformability) of construction materials using similar principles. Rather than "poking" the membrane with a tiny surrogate "finger," I decided to suck the cell membrane into the tip of a micropipette and record the negative pressure required to aspirate the membrane a distance equal to one-half of the diameter (radius) at the open tip.

I made a specialized Barber pipette with a tip opening diameter of ~ 6 microns (~ 0.006 millimeters, mm) and filled it with artificial plasma. The procedure was performed at 400x magnification on the stage of an inverted microscope. The edge of a cell was pulled into the pipette until it reached a distance equal to the radius of the pipette opening (~ 3 microns). The negative pressure in mm H_2O required to cause a hemispherical deformation was dubbed the deformability, a measure of the cell's membrane stiffness. Because vasopressin contracted smooth muscle fibers, in the working hypothesis I had predicted that the hormone would "stiffen" the membrane, requiring a higher pressure to deform it than in cells that were not treated.

Bias is the scientist's worst enemy, especially when the scientist is manually adjusting the pressure device to meet a deformation target and is anxious to chalk up his first independent research effort. So I enlisted my secretary, Alice Dworczack, a new college graduate and wife of medical student David Dworczack, to come to the lab and add the vasopressin to one of two vials of incubation medium labeled A or B while Patti and I were in another room; she added the simple medium to the other vial as a control. Alice wrote the letter of the vial containing the vasopressin on a notepad that she took back to the office. Patti and I would do the studies, measuring the deformability of collecting duct cells alternatively in medium A and B. As a further control, we did the same study in cells from proximal tubules that have no receptors for vasopressin that increase water reabsorption.

When we completed the measurements, we summoned Alice to the lab where Patti would write down the average deformability of the cells in vials A and B. The good news is that in collecting duct cells, we found a big difference in deformability in 10 consecutive experiments; by contrast, in proximal tubule cells deformability was not different between A and B. We had produced the first physical evidence that a reorganization or conformational change occurred in the apical membrane structure of collecting duct cells, the same cellular locus in which vasopressin increased the permeability to water.

The sort of bad news was that I had predicted that the membrane would "harden" or get stiffer in response to vasopressin as proteins within the cells contracted. Our results indicated otherwise; the membrane became more deformable or softer. Fortunately, this was an experiment scientist's dream because any clear-cut result is considered interesting. I concluded that the increase in surface deformability was probably connected to the increased flow of water through the apex of the cells in response to vasopressin. The manuscript describing the first known hormone-induced physical change in a membrane limiting water absorption was published in the esteemed journal "Science" after only minor revision.

I was thrilled by the publication of my first completely independent piece of work in a top science journal — but I soon learned that when you swim alone in a race there is no constituency to cheer or boo when you reach the finish line. I was crestfallen when the abstract of the work I had submitted to the American Society of Nephrology was rejected for presentation at the forth-coming annual meeting. Unfortunately, I had produced an experimental result that no one understood and for which molecular techniques required for deeper investigation would not be available for decades.

But I managed to have some fun with deformability. I was invited to

Yale University to take part in a symposium sponsored by the Department of Physiology in which my Viennese hero, Gerhard Giebisch, had recently become a Professor. This would be my first venture as an independent investigator on a national stage as a competing scientist, and I decided to present the deformability story, which was about to be published in "Science." Moe Burg, Jack Orloff and Bob Berliner would be attending as well. Jack Orloff, for whom I had conflicting feelings, was very outspoken in national meetings or around a lunch table, and I expected that he would make his "stage whisper" comments when my time came to present the deformability story. The time came for my talk, and I took my place at the lectern with Jack sitting in the front row of the amphitheater about 15 feet in front of me. I set up the research question the experiments were intended to address and then explained the procedure in the usual dry scientific lingo.

"We aspirated an apical cap of plasma membrane into the tip of a micropipette that was approximately 6 microns in diameter. The pressure required to suck the membrane a distance equal to the internal radius of the pipette was taken as the deformability. We refer to these as our 'sucking experiments;' they are based on the *Orloff Principle.*" I paused, and after a brief silence, the room exploded in laughter, including Jack. Still smiling, he waved his fist at me in mock anger mouthing, "I'll get even," although he said nothing during my talk or in the discussion that followed. Later, we had a good laugh together over a beer.

The molecular basis underlying the decrease in deformability after treatment with vasopressin was eventually explicated when Peter Agre, M.D. reported that the proteins he discovered and named *aquaporins* formed water pores in the plasma membrane, a finding that earned him the Nobel Prize in 2003. Aquaporins, water channels or pores, in the apical plasma membrane and in tiny vesicles adjacent to it are recycled by trafficking mechanisms that utilize microtubules and microfilaments, the so-called "mini-muscles" I had postulated to be involved in the increased permeability to water. Implantation of the aquaporins evidently changed the physical organization of microfilaments, microtubules and water pores in and about the apex of the cell sufficient to reduce membrane stiffness.

I had to wait four decades before our deformability result was confirmed in collecting duct cells. There is irony here, for so often in science a "novel" American discovery has been reported only to learn that a German scientist had made the same observation half a century before working in a dusty basement laboratory and using primitive tools. Here the geographical table was turned. Riethmuller and colleagues used cutting-edge immunohistochemistry and an even more intimidating method called atomic force microscopy to demonstrate that vasopressin-treated collecting duct cells can be expected to lose rigidity (become more deformable) owing to the relaxation of actomyosin (Biophysical Journal 94:671-678, 2008). Sadly, the published report did not mention our 1970 paper, so I sent a polite "for your information" email and a copy of the "Science" paper to Prof. Riethmuller in Germany and received a prompt apology for the oversight. Moreover, in his next published paper, "Nanotechnology" 21:1-7, 2010, Prof. Riethmuller graciously included the following sentence in the acknowledgements section: "This manuscript is dedicated to Dr. Jared Grantham, whose report about cellular contraction in 1970 is greatly appreciated." Riethmuller's collegial interaction and respect trumped the disappointment that my first "ugly baby" publication garnered in the renal community.

Darryl Fanestil announced late in 1969 that he had accepted a position at the University of California, San Diego and would be leaving KU at the end of the academic year. This was a heavy blow coming on the heels of our recent move, and it was not assuaged by Darryl's offer to take me along with him. Carol and I had no interest in another move coming so soon, even to a location considered paradise by many. Dennis Diederich, Donald Tucker and I huddled and swore allegiance; at least until a new division director was appointed.

A week had not passed before Clifford Gurney, the new chairman of Internal Medicine, called me to his office and asked if I was interested in becoming the next nephrology division director. I responded that I had not thought much about it, as I was still a neophyte and just getting my research program established. He suggested that I think about it and if I was interested, put some goals together we could discuss. Carol and I thought it over for several days and agreed that it might be better to have some authority as I built my research program and nephrology practice than risk being led by a director without a strong academic agenda. I put together a long-term plan for nephrology development that included more faculty and fellowship positions, startup funds for research, improvements in dialysis hardware and enhancements to our renal transplant program with the goal of making Kansas University Nephrology a national leader within two decades. Gurney and I visited again; he read the plan and offered me the position, which I accepted.

Not having done this before, I was pretty naïve about how things really work in the academy. First of all, only fools put together long-term plans or make promises they are not certain they can keep. Things change so rapidly that long-term to most old hands means more than an hour. I imagine that Gurney had a good laugh when I left his office without asking for my recruitment package to be written down, signed and notarized or for my salary to be embellished in the light of the extra work I had just agreed to. Fortunately, there were two solid physician scientists in the division who could be depended on to provide outstanding clinical care and competent teaching while supporting the research goals. Each of us believed that there wasn't anything we could not accomplish if we just worked a little harder — a principle with which our wives probably took exception.

During that first year, Carol got our children enrolled in elementary school or otherwise engaged as she organized our home, found a Methodist Church for us to attend and skillfully kept me engaged in home life while on the run. With only three staff nephrologists and renal programs at KUMC and the Kansas City Veterans hospital to oversee, time became the most precious commodity and time management a survival skill. Upon the advice of Dan Scarpelli, chairman of Pathology, I welcomed Larry Welling, M.D. to the lab as a graduate student seeking a Ph.D. Larry was a very bright and technically-skilled student who also made gorgeous solid oak and walnut furniture in his free time, evidence of the patience and dexterity required to dissect and perfuse tubules. He quickly warmed to the study of isolated perfused tubules, and together we developed a project to determine the tensile properties and the permeability to proteins of tubule basement membranes, the "sausage-casing-like" nets that encircle the cells of a renal tubule. Very quickly, Larry was doing studies on his own as was Patti Qualizza, freeing up more of my time for patient care, teaching and administrative duties.

Fred Whittier, M.D. joined the nephrology division from Vanderbilt and took over as chief of nephrology at the Kansas City Veterans Hospital. A man of high energy and vision, Fred changed the sleepy VA into an exciting post that complemented the activities on the KUMC campus. Within a year, he was joined by Don Cross, M.D. from the University of Missouri, Kansas City who would set up Kansas City's first free-standing tissue typing and organ perfusion laboratory, originally called the Midwest Organ Bank, or MOB for short. The MOB moniker was wholly appropriate as the organization was consummated when tough-minded, competing nephrology leaders from Kansas University, University of Missouri-Kansas City, Kansas City Veterans Hospital and St. Luke's Hospital met at Jimmie's Jigger, a bar on the corner of 39th Street and State Line Road to finalize and approve a "Declaration of Interdependence" I had drafted. That evening, we formulated the name of the organization, The Midwest Organ Bank, a.k.a. the MOB. Over the next 40 years, the name and the location have changed, but the organization is still fiercely interdependent.

In 1971, I was invited to attend a symposium at the Royal College of Physicians in London, all expenses paid for Carol and me. I had attended research meetings, but Carol had always remained at home with the children. This time we would hire a nanny to take care of our children so Carol could see some of the world with me. However, there was one problem. I was expected to present my latest results on the effects of diuretics in kidney tubules, and I had not done any experiments with these drugs.

Most diuretics used to remove swelling about the ankles and lower legs (*edema*) act by decreasing the reabsorption of sodium and chloride by kidney tubules; water is dragged along with the salts, thereby increasing the flow of urine (*diuresis*). The tubule segments where diuretics have their effects had not been clearly identified, so the experiments were worthwhile. If we found that diuretics inhibited fluid absorption in proximal tubules, I would have something unusual to talk about in London.

If we perfused the tubules through and through as we had done at the NIH, we would only be able to do a few experiments each week. Since time was short, I perfused proximal tubules with an open manometer system, rather than a pump, and used the collecting pipette to crimp the other end of the tubule, blocking flow. Consequently, fluid could leave the perfusion pipette only if it was absorbed through the walls of the tubule. I put a droplet of lightweight oil (cigarette lighter fluid, actually) in the shank of the perfusion pipette. As tubules absorbed fluid out of the lumens, the oil drops within the perfusion pipettes moved

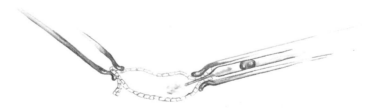

steadily toward the tubules. By recording the rate the oil drop moved along the glass pipette, we could use simple geometry to calculate the volume absorbed per minute, providing a direct readout of the tubule fluid absorption rate. With this set up, Patti could do several experiments each day, giving Carol and me more time to make plans for the trip and purchase our London wardrobes.

Carol found a nice lady to stay with our children while we cavorted about London. It was a delightful experience, a "second honeymoon," but with more coin in our pockets. We met and became lifelong friends with

Saulo and Carol Klahr and Gary and Sibyl Eknoyan, toured Churchill's home at Chartwell and dined at Royal Tunbridge Wells and the Prospect of Whitby. The scientific meeting was a show-and-tell format designed by a pharmaceutical company to launch their new diuretic, zaroxlyn. The invited speakers, considered to be leaders in the world of salt and water metabolism, gave their usual summaries of past research. How I got there and Moe Burg did not is a mystery, but Jack Orloff and Martha Vaughn Orloff's presence led me to notice that only one member of each laboratory appeared to have been invited. I think that my move from NIH may have accelerated my appearance on the world stage of experimental nephrology.

Moe Burg would call me from time to time just to catch up on what I was doing. Our conversations were always friendly and often generated new research insights. If there is a God in heaven, I think he must have been on the line one day when Moe called. I had just returned from London, and I told Moe about the experiments I had done using a modification of his stationary perfusion method, substituting a moving oil droplet for the radioactive water. He complimented me on the clever change to oil — compliments are always hard to get from this guy — but then he raised a concern.

"You know, Jared, the diuretics you are placing in the bath may be secreted into the tubule, build up within the lumen fluid and slow the rate of absorption that way rather than blocking a salt transport mechanism." This is a direct quote because those words were burned into my memory forever. In other words, Moe, the consummate "Devil's advocate," had raised the possibility that the way the diuretics were blocking fluid absorption was unrelated to how I thought they worked.

I don't remember how I responded, but I think I said that he made a good point and that I would test his idea by doing a control experiment using a gold-standard chemical known to be actively secreted into the urine by proximal tubules, the segments I had used for the diuretic experiments. The next afternoon, we repeated the diuretic protocol except that I instructed Patti to put para-aminohippurate (PAH) in the bath rather than a diuretic. I predicted that it would have a minor impact, if any effect at all. I moved to the lab next door to work on data analysis. After about 30 minutes, I heard Patti shout from the other room, "Dr. Grantham, you'd better come in here. Something weird is happening!"

I got up and hurried next door, unsure of what I might find. Patti looked up at me then pointed to the tubule perfusion set-up and said, haltingly, "The oil drop's going backward! Backward!"

I was incredulous thinking this young creature might be having a psychotic moment, but she insisted that the drop was moving in the wrong direction as though the tubule was forcing fluid into the pipette rather than the other way around. I tried to calm her down and sat on the stool while looking into a microscope that was aimed at the oil drop. After blinking a couple of times to be sure my vision was clear, I confirmed that, indeed, the oil drop was climbing up the perfusion pipette. "Can't be," I thought to myself. "You can't make water run uphill. There has got to be a mistake somewhere."

I told Patti to make final measurements and set up another tubule. I would go to Dr. Larry Sullivan's lab and get some different PAH. We must have gotten hold of a rotten lot. I returned with fresh PAH. I took over responsibility for making the measurements this time. During the control periods, the oil drop moved toward the tubule as fluid was absorbed, just as it had always done before. Patti then added the PAH to the bath, and within two minutes, the oil drop slowed to a stop and then began to move away from the tubule, up the pipette. Patti's observation was, indeed, correct. The tubule was secreting fluid into the lumen, evidently linked to the secretion of relatively large amounts of PAH.

I turned the measurements over to Patti and returned to the station where the tubules had been dissected earlier in the day. The tissue was kept chilled and oxygenated, so more than likely extra-dissected tubules would still be viable. It had occurred to me that if we were observing real fluid secretion linked to the secretion of a relatively large anion like PAH, that the lumens of tubules floating freely in a dish should open widely without being perfused at all. I transferred the tubules into a 37 degree centigrade incubation chamber on the stage of an inverted microscope filled with medium containing PAH and watched them intensely at 400x magnification. Miraculously, after two minutes, the lumens, which ordinarily are totally collapsed after removing the tissue from its blood supply, began to show a slight crack where the lumens would be expected. Within 10 minutes, the lumens of several tubules were widely distended proving that PAH provoked the secretion of fluid into the tubule lumen.

In an afternoon, we had discovered and proven — by accident — that proximal renal tubules can secrete fluid into the lumen coupled to the transport of PAH! This was a novel and surprising result because the "kidney Gods" at the NIH, New York City, New Haven and Boston held that well-intentioned renal tubules did not secrete fluid like lower caste tear ducts, sweat glands and intestines.

I tried desperately to imagine what this new finding meant in the overall scheme of renal function and could not generate even a bad idea. Without a strong rationale to dress up this bizarre new function, I risked being jeered by those in the upper circle of renal physiology who, until then, had seemed to be lifting me into higher standing. In 1972, it was widely believed that renal tubules absorbed salt and water — about 99 percent of what the glomeruli filtered was absorbed back into the blood — leaving about 1 percent left over to be excreted as urine. There were well-known tubule transport mechanisms to secrete acid, potassium, hippurates and other organic flotsam — but not fluid! The canon held that the human kidney filters and reabsorbs fluid — period!

Throughout my life, there had been moments that in sum led me to believe that I was on a providential journey; the sudden and rather bizarre events of the day signaled that my voyage had reached a major turning point. Later in the quiet of the night after I had made water run uphill, I continued to wrestle with the ecstasy of discovery and the torment of potential professional ruination. Then, in some remote cloister of my brain, Ronnie Wilkerson's polycystic kidneys collided with Ken Gardner's seminal discovery reported in the 1969 "New England Journal of Medicine." Gardner had analyzed the composition of cyst fluids from a single polycystic kidney and concluded that renal cysts were giant renal tubules that continued to function like the nephron segments from which they derived, even in patients whose overall renal function had reached end-stage.

I had learned in medical school that polycystic kidneys were rather grotesque structures that leave a firm imprint in one's memory the first time they are seen at an operation or autopsy (Figure, polycystic and normal kidneys). The kidneys are stuffed with individual fluid-filled sacs developing within microscopic renal tubules that enlarge progressively over the patient's lifetime. Kidneys that normally weigh less than a pound are known to weigh more than 20 pounds in the fully-developed condition, causing marked protrusion of the abdomen and giving the owner a configuration often referred to as a "beer belly." The innumerable cysts crowd out the normal tissue and eventually cause renal failure in the fifth and sixth decades in most patients. Gardner had sampled and analyzed the fluids in only a single case of PKD, an afternoon's work that was rewarded by a publication in one of the world's most influential medical journals.

Earlier than usual the next morning, I drove to work above the legal limits prepared to develop and explore a new hypothesis of renal cyst formation and expansion.

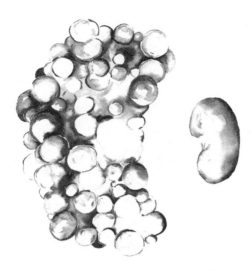

Normal kidney (right) and polycystic kidney (left). Individuals would have two normal or two polycystic kidneys. The normal kidney is about the size of a human hand. The polycystic kidney is greatly enlarged by cysts of different sizes, all of which began in renal tubules about the size of a hair on the back of your hand.

❖

CHAPTER 24

A time to reflect

My brain was a tangle of thoughts as the unexpected discovery of fluid secretion spun about seeking deeper understanding in PKD. I captured one idea and wrote it down before the thought evaporated. Years earlier, an anonymous substance, discovered in the blood of all patients with extreme kidney failure, was found to block the renal excretion of hippurate, a normal product of metabolism. Hippurate and PAH, the stuff that made water run uphill the day before, were similar chemicals, so perhaps the aberrant substance retained in kidney failure might make kidney cysts enlarge by stimulating the secretion of fluid into them. The blood dialysis unit was just a few steps from my lab and clotted blood, used to determine the bleeding time of anti-coagulated patients, was there for the taking. I collected a few small tubes and separated the serum from the red blood cells. I took some of Patti's freshly dissected kidney tubules left over in the dish from the morning experiment and put them into medium supplemented with human serum from the dialysis unit. I incubated the tubules for 10 minutes at body temperature and then examined them in the high-powered microscope. The lumen of every proximal tubule was widely distended with fluid! This meant that a chemical, resembling the PAH we had used in the crucial experiments the day before, must be present in the blood of patients with renal failure at levels much higher than normal.

Today, rapidly connecting the dots as I had just done would be considered highly unethical and illegal. I had no formal protocol certified by the Institutional Review Board (IRB) for this particular foray into clinical investigation; I took a patient's blood without seeking signed, informed permission from the patient, even though the tube of clotted blood was unidentified and scheduled for discard; I introduced human blood into a laboratory research setting without having taken a course on workplace safety and passing a certifying test. In other words, my inspired moment of insight and immediate reward would not happen today unless I jumped through all of the institutional hoops that usually take four to eight weeks to gain approval before I could give it a try. Consequently, inspired moments such as this one are rarely attempted anymore because they don't usually turn up anything positive or conclusive and the invested research time in preparing all of the paperwork is wasted.

I settled on a two-pronged attack on PKD: One, I would devote a significant portion of the lab effort on studies to flush out the nature of the secretion-causing chemical in the blood of patients with kidney failure, and two, I would start collecting as many polycystic kidneys discarded as surgical specimens as I could find in order to review in greater detail the physiologic, anatomic and pathologic changes that go on within kidneys as they develop the cysts that ultimately cause the function of the organ to fail.

There was also excitement on the clinical side of my career. Clifford Gurney resigned as chairman of the Department of Internal Medicine, and Norton Greenberger, M.D., a "fire-breathing" gastroenterologist from Ohio State, was hired to replace him. Greenberger promised that he would make KU Internal Medicine the Midwest equivalent of Harvard medicine. He was culture shock to many on our faculty with blank academic resumes, and they sought refuge elsewhere. He was heaven's manna for me as we spoke the same academic language as those in leading academic organizations for internists and other physician scientists that counted us as members. He helped me recruit Arnold Chonko, M.D., a graduate of Ohio State School of Medicine and All-American football defenseman during Woody Hayes' glory years. Arnie joined as a laboratory research fellow and two years later became an Assistant Professor of Internal Medicine in the Nephrology Division. Students and residents in Internal Medicine were attracted to Arnie's manner of teaching at the bedside like June bugs to a porch light. They knew an outstanding physician when they saw one, but in addition, he mesmerized those under his watch with anecdotes and stories of patients and their maladies. Arnie also developed a micro-perfusion lab, like mine, where he did some landmark work on the renal excretion of hippurate and uric acid, the chemical that causes gout.

A year later, Virginia Savin, M.D. joined our group from the University of Washington where she had trained with Belding Scribner, the man who developed chronic blood dialysis and peritoneal dialysis used to treat patients with irreversible kidney failure. Virginia, an intellectually gifted and compassionate physician, introduced peritoneal dialysis to the program. She had done some laboratory training as a renal fellow but was relatively untested as an independent researcher when she arrived. I set her up in a laboratory with a research assistant to do some studies on glomeruli, the tuft of blood vessels that become inflamed in "Bright's Disease," otherwise known as *glomerulonephritis*. The million or so glomeruli at the beginning of each nephron are responsible for generating about 40 gallons of urine each day from blood passing through the kidneys. Within a year, she had developed a unique method for quantifying the filtration properties of individual glomeruli isolated from kidneys and maintained in an artificial environment. She would use this new method to discover a novel substance in blood plasma that causes severe damage to glomeruli and loss of kidney function in patients.

Mike Linshaw, M.D. joined the renal group to create a Division of Pediatric Nephrology. He spent the first year as a faculty member working in my laboratory, determining how individual renal tubules regulate their cell volumes, before launching his independent research career. A gifted experimentalist, Mike was also an outstanding bedside pediatric physician. He had an uncanny knack for solving the most complex problems that affect children, a talent that was widely recognized among academic pediatric nephrologists.

The extra help provided by these remarkable colleagues gave me more time to think about urine. In a trip to the library, I had learned that cranberries and prunes contained an abundance of quinic acid, a precursor of hippurate. If the fluid-secretion-provoking substance in uremic serum was a hippurate-like molecule, I thought it might show up in the serum and urine of normal persons eating relatively large amounts of cranberries and prunes. I was anxious to test this hypothesis and was fortunate to recruit Robert Porter, M.D., one of our star nephrology fellows, and a medical student, William Cathcart-Rake, to participate in a short-term clinical trial — on us. There were no informed consent mavens lurking in the halls to prevent us from doing research on ourselves. Moreover, the three of us "volunteered" our wives to participate as well. We all ate a bland, organic diet, concocted by dietician Pat Stein, for several days, then heaping helpings of prunes or cranberries were added for several more days. We collected our urine daily and drew blood samples at the beginning and the end of the study. We developed a simple bioassay to determine if the mystery factor appeared in the blood and urine.

After one day on the diet, Joan Porter had a severe migraine attack precipitated by the sudden withdrawal from caffeine required by the study protocol. Thankfully, the experiment proved highly successful, minus one transiently-disabled caffeine addict; 40 years later, she and I remain friends. This study is still mentioned in some circles as the "prune trial." Jerry Cohlmia, M.D., a clinical nephrology fellow and neophyte laboratory researcher, set up a chemical assay for hippurate while leaving sulfuric acid burns on a large surface of the laboratory bench where he worked — a place he has been known to visit on Alumni Day. His analysis showed that the secretory substance in the blood of patients with kidney failure was hippurate and that it could be removed by hemodialysis.

I decided to extend the pioneering work of Ken Gardner and Andrew Evan and test the idea that renal cysts were in fact overgrown tubules that had become fluid-filled, tumor-like masses. It is not unusual for painful or unusually large polycystic kidneys to be surgically removed. I had collected several of these discarded specimens, collected and stored the fluids within the cysts and preserved the tissue for high-resolution anatomic study. Francis Cuppage, M.D., a nephro-pathologist, used sophisticated electron microscopy techniques to define the cellular structure of renal cysts, and Richard Huseman, M.D., a renal fellow, analyzed the chemical content of cyst fluid. This team gave us the anatomic facts we needed to construct hypotheses about the formation and sustained growth of renal cysts.

After seven years at KUMC, I was eligible for a sabbatical leave, an important fringe benefit of academic life offered to faculty to keep their science competitive. I chatted with my former division director, Darrell Fanestil, about places to go and he suggested Cambridge University, where he and his family were headed for a year. I found a place in Ian Glynn's laboratory where I could work on aspects of the sodium pump, the major energy-consuming enzyme in the kidney.

Ian Glynn, M.D., a physician scientist and a Fellow of Trinity College, performed formative studies to clarify the mechanisms by which the sodium pump exchanged sodium for potassium across biological membranes. I had friends at Yale who had worked with Glynn when he spent time there during his own sabbatical leave in the United States; they helped sneak me into Cambridge without Ian detecting beforehand that he would be hosting an ignoramus. I arranged for a renal laboratory research fellow, Jim Irish, Ph.D., M.D., and Rich Huseman to keep things humming in the lab while I was away. Alice and David Dworzack rented our house (and cat). Carol packed everything each of us would need for the next nine months into suitcases and duffel bags, and the six of us took flight to Cambridge.

With the help of Ian's wife, Jennifer, I had arranged with a real estate firm to let a house in Cambridge, only to discover a week before we were to arrive that the owner had decided to not leave town. Jennifer went back to work and found another place in the village of Toft, just 6 miles west of Cambridge. However, on the day we pulled into Cambridge in two cars I had hired beforehand to meet us at Heathrow Airport, we learned from the real estate agent that the house in Toft was no longer available and that we would be put up in two college housing units until something could be found. Taylor, Aaron, Joel and I stayed in one apartment and Carol and Janeane in another about two blocks away. We had no bedclothes, bathroom towels or kitchen gear. Located on the outskirts of Cambridge without a means of transportation, we felt like scruffy, unwelcome immigrants in a foreign land. We found a pub that had edible food and filled our hungry bellies, then lay down on bare mattresses in our respective quarters and slept soundly in the summer warmth for the next 10 or 12 hours.

The next morning, I walked a couple of miles to a Barclay's Bank in the center of Cambridge where I planned to set up a checking account using a certified check in pounds sterling I had gotten from a correspondent bank in the United States. But alas, the bank encounter did not go smoothly as the teller believed that I could not draw any money from my new account until the check had "cleared," a process that would take a week. I had enough cash for us to get along, but I needed to buy a car and needed access to the larger sum tied up in the certified check. I should have suspected that this bank was not up to speed when I noticed, while standing in queue, that tellers serving other customers were using pencils and paper to do simple addition and subtraction in the course of making deposits or withdrawals. There were no adding machines in sight.

I protested loudly that I had used a correspondent bank in the United States to avoid a delay in the transfer of funds and demanded to speak to his supervisor. After meeting and forcefully making my case to that supervisor, I was finally escorted to see another higher-ordered Pooh-bah who finally gave in to my request. With checkbook in hand, I walked another two miles to an automobile dealership on the outskirts of Cambridge. Within an hour, I had purchased a Volvo station wagon with the understanding that they would buy it back from me in nine months for what I paid minus 500 pounds. Having contacted the AAA and my U.S. insurer before leaving home, I was armed with an international driver's license and insurance coverage as I drove out of the auto dealership, struggling to not drift over to the right side of the road.

My waiting family was favorably impressed with our new means of transportation. The real estate agent had found more hospitable housing on Maid's Causeway that would be available in a few days for a period not longer than three weeks, giving us a place to get grounded until we found a more permanent location. We had a few days to burn before moving to Maids Causeway, so we decided to break out of the antiquated college housing and make a quick run to the north, passing through our ancestral home of Grantham on our way to Scotland, staying in bed and breakfast inns along the way.

My uncle Don Grantham was stationed in England during World War II and had made a trip to Grantham to see if any relatives might remain in the town. I was in the fourth grade when he told me about his grand trip to Grantham, which is about 100 miles north of London on the Great North Road in the midlands. After getting off the train in his Army uniform, he walked about a mile into town down a street lined by single-family houses on either side. On the front porch of one of the houses, an old man smoking a pipe rocked his chair back and forth as Uncle Don strolled by. My uncle said that the man called to him to come up to the porch so that he could get a better look at him.

"You must be a Grantham, you look just like 'em," the old man exclaimed, according to my uncle Don.

That's as much as I can remember of my Army hero's story, but at my impressionable age, just imagining there was a whole town that resembled my descendants was permanently embedded in my cerebral cortex. I had repeated Uncle Don's storied trip to Grantham dozens of times to anyone who would listen and especially my own children. As we pulled into the outskirts of Grantham, Aaron spoke out from the back section of the station wagon, where he was usually banished along with Taylor.

"Gee, Dad. Do you think they'll recognize us?"

"We'll soon find out," I replied.

I stopped at an intersection to gather my bearings, and before I knew it, Carol had hopped out of the car and into a red phone booth. I could see her rustling through the book, wildly flipping through the white and yellow pages. She had heard my "Uncle Don" story so many times she was as anxious as anyone to get some hard data before getting back into the car.

"Jared," she said sardonically, "there are no, N-O, Granthams in Grantham."

I got out and confirmed her finding. Dang! Uncle Don had perpetuated a myth that I had taken as gospel for years. This misadventure was just another notch on my "Sucker Belt of Naivety." We walked about Grantham, cornering any of the locals who would speak to us, trying to shed some light on the absence of Granthams in Grantham. We were received politely, but it soon became evident that the town's citizens didn't care a twit about who the Granthams were. On the other hand, they were quick to brag on Isaac Newton and Margaret Thatcher who were born and raised there.

Grantham has suffered from more than the abdications of those who bear its name. The Great North Road once ran through the center of the town, creating an environment for robust trade and industry. That ended when the city fathers built a highway to divert the traffic and tore down nearly all of the historic buildings lining the main street. Sadly, I must confess that the year after we returned to Kansas, the London Times feted Grantham as "The most boring city in England."

But losers sometimes have their day. There currently circulates a new and more compelling myth than even my uncle Don could dream up. The public television series "Downton Abbey" has surged into our living rooms with record-breaking numbers of viewers and critical acclaim. It takes place in Yorkshire in the early 20th century, and guess what, one of the leading characters, Lord Grantham, is the keeper of the estate. And you know, I think I bear a physical resemblance.

The remainder of the trip was a feast of Roman Ruins, cathedrals, estate houses and emerald green countryside punctuated with lakes famed by poetry and monsters. We returned to Cambridge ready to settle down and become more gentrified. The real estate agent had come up with another potential house in Toft, not far from the earlier one we had lost. Named Priory Cottage, the house was a block from an Anglican church on a narrow country lane and partially concealed behind a living fence. Portions had been built before the pilgrims sailed to America and the "newer" rooms, added within the last 100 years, were constructed of heavy, polished timber. An oil-fired furnace and electric heaters that came on when the rates were low provided heat, meaning that we would need to dress in layers during the winter. This would be an idyllic place to live; a large living-room window framed a John Constable landscape of green pastures, blackberry-laden fences and contented sheep and cattle grazing peacefully throughout the day.

We had only one more hurdle to jump. The house served as the summer cottage for Sir Donald Tebbit, the British Ambassador to Australia, and his wife, Lady Tebbit. Lady Tebbit had asked to meet our entire family for tea, after which she would decide whether or not to rent the house to us. Carol had dressed the children carefully and removed most of the dirt from the arms and under the fingernails of our three very active sons. I had lectured to them as well about good behavior and courtesy. We sat with Lady Tebbit and had our tea — I even refrained from dunking the biscuits. We chitchatted for several minutes, and then she said we could have the house provided we would look after her two free-range cats that were out hunting at the time. We shook hands on the deal and left in triumph, prepared to move in after two weeks.

Thus began, perhaps, the most cherished year in the life of our little family. We were together and reliant on one another in an exotic paradise free from the constraints of the workplace. The children were happy in their new schools where their sharp Kansas speech stood out against the consonant-less sounds made by British children. Carol could expect me to come home at a decent hour of the day and she could organize family outings nearly every weekend along with three longer trips to the continent.

My parents and sister, Annetta, visited; for them, this was the greatest adventure of their lifetime. My father had the ruddy physical attributes of English men and fit right in when he snuck off to the neighborhood pub for a pinter. I took a week off to show them the sights of London and the English countryside. My mother had seen enough "musty old castles and churches" after a day trip to the white cliffs of Dover. During our London visit, we ate dinner at the Swiss Centre where they served outstanding cheese fondue along with delicious white wine. After dinner, Annie lit a cigarette, and I decided I would have one as well, as I had been on the wagon for several months. I got to take one puff before Janeane and her brothers began crying loudly, compelling all eyes in the restaurant to look our way as I sheepishly snubbed out my guilty pleasure.

My project in the Glynn lab at Downing Site was to characterize the effects of vanadate on the sodium pump. Vanadate, a mineral first-cousin of phosphate, is found in normal tissue and bone in trace amounts. Its role in physiologic processes was unknown. Over the nine-month assignment, I completed three projects with lots of help from Ian Glynn, Jose Cavieres, Ken Rubinson and William Balfour. It was a great learning experience for me, as I attended lectures by outstanding scientists at Cambridge and visitors from around the world. Ian was a gracious host who did not get upset when I messed up my first experiment on red blood cells or confessed that I had not read all of Jane Austen's novels. I had not worked in the lab at home for a couple of years, leaving that to technicians and research fellows, so I was a bit of a pig in the lab for a week or two. But I finally found my groove and began getting useful results.

The new science I was desperately trying to comprehend and participate in meaningfully helped to clear some of the cobwebs in my brain leftover from Kansas. But still in bondage, I couldn't quit thinking about urine altogether. We were studying the mechanisms by which vanadate blocked the action of the sodium pump in human red blood cells. It was very powerful stuff. Because kidney tubules use the sodium pump to reclaim those 40 gallons of salt water filtered by the glomeruli, it occurred to me that vanadate might turn out to be a strong diuretic, i.e. increase urine flow and salt excretion with it. Ian had spent his entire career working with red blood cells and was not especially fond of the kidney. Nonetheless, he recruited William Balfour, a member of the Physiology Department with a vivi-section license, to collaborate with us to determine if vanadate had diuretic properties. When we infused sodium vanadate into a conscious rat, there followed an immense increase in urine flow, reflecting the effect of the molecule to inhibit the reabsorption of sodium in renal tubules. A short paper describing the mechanism of diuresis caused by vanadate was accepted for publication by "Nature," a premier British science journal.

While in Cambridge, I met and collaborated with Jose Cavieres, Ph.D., a fellow in Ian's lab. We did not hit it off at first. Jose was a Chilean expatriate who was forced out of his country when the ruthless Augusto Pinochet overthrew Salvador Allende. Jose blamed the American CIA for his country's debacle and held me personally responsible. He believed that in a democracy, individual citizens had a say in such things. When he settled down enough to learn that I wasn't even sure where Chile was and did not know the names of the current or past leaders, he was finally persuaded that I was too ignorant to be considered an enemy. Before my term ended at Cambridge, we shared authorship on a publication and became good friends.

Our sabbatical abroad brought our family closer together and provided fodder for endearing memories that will last a lifetime. Moreover, Carol and I learned that two shy, stay-at-home Kansans had become proficient at packing up our children and charging off across a vast expanse without a home to greet us on arrival, just so I could think about urine.

CHAPTER 25

Romancing the cyst with Mr. Joseph H. Bruening

The anatomic studies I was doing in collaboration with Francis Cuppage were paying off handsomely. In cysts with diameters slightly larger than the tubules in which they formed (0.1 millimeters) and ranging to more than 60 millimeters, we observed minute anatomic details at magnifications 10,000 greater than the targeted objects. We proved that cysts were lined by a single layer of cells, called an *epithelium*, that were joined together by "tight" junctions functioning like "spot welds" around the top of each cell.

Kidney tubules can be thought of as a garden hose in which the wall is made of individual cells welded together at the top to form a tube-like structure surrounding a central cavity (*lumen*) usually full of urine. A six-pack of beer held together at the top by a plastic wrap is a good anatomic model of the individual cells (beer cans) sealed together to prevent the leakage of fluid or certain molecules between the cells. Cells held together this way are called *epithelia*. Kidney tubules are in fact tiny hoses about the same size as human hair. The epithelial lining effectively seals the tubule, keeping the liquid in the lumen (*urine*) from mixing with fluids bathing the outside of the cells (*interstitium*). Renal cysts are simply very large tubules that trap fluid within an expanding cavity lined by epithelium. Rich Huseman's analysis of mineral and acid profiles in dozens of cysts from several kidneys confirmed Ken Gardner's finding in a single polycystic kidney.

We also observed that the thin basement membranes around normal tubules were piled up around cysts like growth rings in a tree stump; there was a buildup of inflammatory cells and scar tissue outside the cysts as well. Frank Carone, M.D. had made similar observations in Chicago. Clearly, cysts were greatly expanded renal tubules that were composed of epithelial cells; however, the total number of cells lining the walls of expanded cysts were often hundreds of times more numerous than the tubules from which they derived. In other words, the growth of cells within the cysts appeared to have something to do with causing the walls to expand.

Andrew Evan, Ph.D. and Jay Bernstein, M.D. were the first to recognize that the vastly increased number of cells within cysts sometimes led to the formation of polyps that would project from the wall. The technical term for this excessive cellular growth is *proliferation*. Our work provided unequivocal confirmation that each cyst was a product of increased cell growth. We now had evidence from several laboratories that cysts were unusual neoplasms (*tumors*) in which the largest mass is the fluid within the cavity filling the space created by the ever-expanding wall. It is important to note that the *neoplasia* (new growth) featured in cysts is not malignant, i.e. the cells do not spread to other parts of the body. Serious cancers can develop in polycystic kidneys, but the occurrence rate is no greater than in the population at large.

The profound changes we saw in the basement membranes surrounding each cyst interested a KUMC colleague, Billy Hudson, Ph.D., who was analyzing the chemical structure of these basement membranes in glomerular diseases including diabetes mellitus. An internationally known biochemist, Hudson approached me about a collaboration that I joyfully embraced. Together we would try to determine if the abnormalities in the basement membranes of cysts were a reflection of the aberrant genetic machinery passed from parent to child in the families of PKD patients. We obviously needed more clinical material to address these new science opportunities with improved analytical methods that were certain to come along.

I started a PKD clinic and quickly accumulated several dozen patients, all of whom were anxious to learn more about their disease and the mode of inheritance. Little was known about the genetics or how cysts form and harm the kidneys, and we were eager to learn as much about the pathophysiology of the disease as current methods would allow. There were only five or six laboratories in the world interested in research of PKD. Sadly, a new textbook of Nephrology edited by two outstanding scientists failed to include a chapter or even mention PKD. When asked to speak about PKD research, which wasn't often, I usually began the lecture by referring to it as a "Dangerfield Disorder," in tribute to comedian Rodney Dangerfield whose standup act was built around his oft-repeated complaint, "I don't get any respect!"

In my "act" before medical audiences, I would confidently blurt out in defense, "Cysts are, without question, the most important cellular structures in biology!" as a photograph of several isolated cyst-like structures was being projected onto the screen at the front of the room.

"And what kind of cysts are these?" I would ask.

Invariably, the audience would answer, "Kidney cysts."

"No!" I would snort with mock disgust.

"These are blastocysts" (*a multi-cell stage of the embryo following conception*). "Think about this. Everyone in this room was once a blasto-CYST, although most of you have advanced to a higher state of differentiation."

This opening was usually sufficient to keep them awake a few minutes longer.

Computed tomography scans had just become clinically available and together with radiologist Errol Levine, M.D., I was able to gather more objective information about each patient's experience with pain, urinary tract hemorrhage, kidney stones and renal failure. We also studied a large number of patients with diseases other than hereditary PKD who, nonetheless, developed cysts within the kidneys as the underlying disease progressed to the end stage. This is a secondary condition called *acquired renal cystic disease*. In the acquired forms of renal cystic disease, the incidence of cancer is approximately 40 times greater than in the inherited disorders.

I continued to explore the role of organic anions like hippurate in the promotion of cyst growth, but that trail was growing colder by the day. The levels of hippurate we measured in the cyst fluids were much too low to account for the amount of fluid that had accumulated within them. I suspected that fluid secretion had a role to play, but it was becoming painfully clear that hippurate was the wrong suspect. We continued to discover bits and pieces of useful information in the lab about the anatomy and pathology of cystic kidneys, and we had a growing cohort of patients in whom computed tomography scans were providing important information about disease progression. But we were years away from making a meaningful impact with so few scientists in the world working on the problem. I had often wondered what it would take to stir up the scientific and lay community's interest in PKD. I was about to find out.

One day late in 1980, I was sitting in the lab looking over some data when a young woman I did not know walked in and introduced herself. She was Kathleen Fisher, the medical writer for the city's major newspaper, The Kansas City Star. She was on campus looking for interesting medical stories and had been sent from the Dean's office to see me. We engaged in the usual light talk. Then she asked me to tell her what I was doing in the lab. She seemed to have time on her hands, so I began the long version of the tale about the third most common cause of kidney failure in the world and how little was known about it. I emphasized its genetic basis and that it was more common than cystic fibrosis, sickle cell anemia and muscular dystrophy — all better known than PKD with hundreds of research scientists working on the problems enjoying strong support from the NIH. As far as I knew, there was only one active PKD grant funded by the NIH — mine.

She inquired about what cysts were, and I walked her through a quick course in renal physiology. Medical writers in that day were well-trained and highly informed, so not much time was needed to bring her to a relatively high level of understanding. I explained the two prevalent hypothesis of cyst formation — obstruction of tubule urine flow by over-grown polyps (Gardner and Evan) and weakness in the tubule basement membrane (Grantham, Hudson and Carone) — neither of which proved to be the case, by the way. She stayed for at least two hours and seemed genuinely impressed with what I had to say.

Her last words as she left the lab were, "I'll write you a good story, Dr. Grantham."

I had no idea when the story might run. After a month of diligently scanning The Star, I gave up. Word drifted to me through a channel I can't recall that Ms. Fisher had left the newspaper.

"Well, must have been the cyst story that did her in," I thought to myself.

The New Year came, January passed, and still no story appeared. I had given up on ever seeing anything when on Sunday, February 15, 1981, at the top of page 44 in the A section of the newspaper the headline read:

Research Lags On Hereditary Condition, Specialist Says
By Kathleen Fisher

Beneath the bold headline lay a six-column story that faithfully reflected what I had said during the interview months earlier. The article was buried so deeply in the paper, I wondered if an editor had discovered it when cleaning out Fisher's desk and in the desperation of a slow news day had added it as "filler." A few of my colleagues at KUMC saw it, and it was picked up for wider distribution throughout Kansas through the Medical Center's news service. Ronnie Wilkerson, in Johnson City on the western edge of the state and my inspiration to work on PKD, sent me word that he had seen it and was very excited about what I was doing. But the most momentous acknowledgement did not arrive until early December 1981, in a letter typed on expensive, tan paper bearing the business address of Bruening Properties.

In a carefully crafted letter, Joseph H. Bruening, writing from Kansas City, Missori, explained that he had seen the article in the The Star but that business affairs had kept him from contacting me sooner and that he was leaving immediately for Arizona for the winter. He inquired about the possibility of supporting research in polycystic kidney disease. His wife had the disease and there was a good possibility that they would have funds to contribute toward research of the condition. He asked for my suggestions "as to the most effective use of such money and a general idea of the amount needed to create a chance for an effective result."

I had no idea who this man was except that from spring to late fall he lived in a large ranch-style house at 65th Street and State Line Road in the "tony" district of Kansas City, Missouri. Acquaintance Lynwood Smith, M.D., a graduate of the University of Kansas School of Medicine and at the time a staff nephrologist at the Mayo Clinic, had grown up in that part of town. I suspected that a man like Bruening was "checking me out," so why shouldn't I do some due diligence of my own? I called Lyn for an assessment. Lyn told me that Joe came from a respected Kansas City family and was listed among the blue-bloods of Kansas City society. He didn't know much about his business affairs except that he had inherited several major buildings in downtown Kansas City that he had recently sold. Lyn suspected that he had quite a bit of "coin" in his pocket and could afford to do something substantial.

With this information in hand, I promptly crafted my own letter suggesting that he might consider two general options: One, he could lend support to the National Kidney Foundation and encourage them to pay more attention to PKD or start an independent foundation specifically for PKD, or two, he could stimulate research by financially supporting scientists and their programs of study directed at PKD. I pointed out that the money required could range from modest to very large sums, depending on the donor's appetite. I offered to take his phone call or visit with him over lunch when he was in Kansas City.

I since learned that he wanted to keep everything as close to Kansas City as he could so that he might have the enjoyment of watching it grow. In his next letter, he asked me to put together a comprehensive plan for tackling PKD and to attach some risk and benefit estimations to each component. He wanted to take the plan to Kansas City philanthropies and get additional support to match what he would give. I sent him a detailed plan, including risk/benefit estimations, for a large PKD research and clinical evaluation program at KUMC, which he sent cold-turkey to several large foundations in Kansas City whose executive directors he happened to know. Mr. Bruening soon learned that he needed a lot more training in philanthropic development work when he received in return letters littered with friendly, personal and gracious phrases that had been carefully added to soften the blow of rejection. I think he learned from these disappointing encounters that PKD and Kansas University were going to be hard to sell.

We finally met on May 11, 1982, for lunch at the exclusive River Club situated on a bluff high above the Missouri River near where it turns north toward the headwaters in Montana. This meeting would determine if I dressed appropriately, had decent table manners, used proper syntax and had no despicable attributes like picking my nose. I was advised by Bill Ruth, M.D., my friend and former teacher, who had married into elite Kansas City society, that I should do my best to "sparkle." He tried hard to explain what "sparkle" meant in this context, but unfortunately, I found nothing in my dining repertoire or moderately skewed physical carriage that could be polished. I was clean-shaven and bathed regularly — that would have to do.

Joseph Bruening was waiting for me in the club's foyer. We shook hands and introduced ourselves after which I was directed to the lavatory to "wash up" before going into the dining area. Membership in the exclusive River Club is a cherished status symbol for Kansas City businessmen of substantial means. Tom Watson, famous golfer, is a prized member as well as the mayor, former mayors, Federal and State legislators and the lions of industry. The furniture is framed in dark woods and the walls and carpet are dark. Fortunately, the dining room was well lit through large, encircling windows. However, on overcast days, it too is dark. On this, my maiden venture, and visits thereafter, I felt cloistered, as though whispering might be the preferred means of cross-table communication.

The head waiter escorted us to our table. On the way, Mr. Bruening discreetly asked the waiter for the name of a man dining alone at a table next to ours. When we reached our destination, Mr. Bruening reached out to shake hands with the man nearby, addressing him by his first name and then introducing him to me. Thankfully, he had remembered my name. With this sacrament, Joseph Bruening began the unremitting task of mentoring Jared J. Grantham, M.D., unrefined farm hand from Johnson, Kansas, in the fine art of the business lunch and other social encounters in the elite world.

On a later occasion, Mr. Bruening and I were walking together along an airport corridor on our way to catch a flight when he spotted a man approaching us.

"Jared, that man ahead — I've forgotten his name. I'm going to show you how to find it out without giving away my absent-mindedness."

When we reached the oncoming man, Mr. Bruening reached out his hand and said, "I want you to meet Dr. Jared Grantham."

The man extended his right hand toward me and said, "I'm John Doe, and I'm pleased to meet you, Jared. How are you, Joe?"

As the man walked past, Mr. Bruening turned to me and said, "Jared, in business, it's a sin not to address someone you have met previously by their first name." I've done my best ever since not to violate "Bruening's Law."

Once seated, our conversation was a little stilted at first. He was out of his element on topics of medicine and science, and I was in a challenging environment. Each time we got the conversation rolling, a waiter or maître d' would butt in to put a napkin in our lap, recite the menu or fill water glasses we had not touched. Mr. Bruening wanted to know more about the hereditary cause of PKD, about which I could offer only descriptive information, defining the more common dominant form of the disease in contrast to the rare recessive presentation in children. I advised that we should probably focus on the dominant type as it touches more people who would be needed to increase awareness of PKD. I strongly urged him to direct his resources to determine the cause and search for a cure rather than treating the end-stage of the disease. The federal government was already doing that by supporting dialysis and renal transplantation.

It crossed my mind that a life-long Missouri resident who lived on the Missouri side of State Line Road might find it difficult to support a program in Kansas when all of his political clout was in his home state. So I mentioned to Mr. Bruening that he might consider doing something on more of a regional or national basis rather than focusing on a single institution such as KUMC. I reminded him I had included in my first letter to him that he might want to start a freestanding foundation focused on PKD research. A foundation would leverage his personal contributions and capture more persons like him who might want to become proactive on behalf of their families.

I told him I would be pleased to tell him more about my nascent plan to create a PKD Center at KUMC, but it seemed to me that if real progress was to be made in this unexplored area, that he needed a mechanism to get more good scientists working on the problem. That's when I sprung on him the suggestion that he provide start-up funds to bring several PKD researchers together to write a Program Project Grant (PPG) to the National Institutes of Health. In PPGs, the federal government awards relatively large sums of money to a group of scientists to work on a specific disease or disorder. The scientists may all be located in a single institution if the critical mass of scholars is large enough, or as is the case of PKD, researchers with credentials in this unexplored disorder could be scattered about the nation. He listened but did not commit to the plan; rather, he abruptly concluded the meeting by saying that he would be in touch with me as he arose from the table. I learned at that moment that Mr. Bruening did not make hasty decisions.

A few days later, he asked me to stop by his house on State Line

Road to meet his wife, Allene, and to discuss our mutual PKD interests. Mr. Bruening met me at the door and led me to Mrs. Bruening, who was standing near the fireplace in the living room. A handsome, elegantly dressed woman in her 60s with short blond hair, she extended her hand and smiled warmly as she reached for mine while greeting me with a strong voice that identified her as someone used to being heard. I did my best to emit "sparkle," but I think flop sweat popped out instead.

We sat on couches arranged in a U configuration before the fireplace in the large living room of a classical ranch style house decorated in the colors and artifacts of the American southwest. During several minutes of ritual conversation reserved for getting acquainted sessions, I learned that Mr. Bruening's general reticence had probably been conditioned by Mrs. Bruening's assertiveness. Things must have gone well up to this point because Mr. Bruening suddenly interjected something to the effect that now that we were to become partners in a new foundation to cure PKD, why didn't I address them as "Joe" and "Allene" to save words and time. I replied that it would be fine as long as they called me "Jared" and my wife "Carol." We had come to our first agreement, and I had learned, without a formal pronouncement, of their decision to go forward with the foundation.

We chatted a little longer, and then I headed for home. On the way out, Joe told me that he had conferred with his personal attorney, Ilus Davis, former mayor of Kansas City, Missouri, and advised him to put together the articles of incorporation for a not-for-profit medical foundation seeking to cure PKD. Joe wanted to talk more with me about the structure of the foundation and the possibility of sponsoring a multi-institutional Program Project Grant. This was both wonderful and troubling news, for I would be leaving Kansas City in two weeks to look at a faculty leadership position at Vanderbilt University.

A year earlier, I had strayed away from Kansas to visit Yale University in response to an invitation from Sam Thier, M.D., chairman of the Department of Internal Medicine. He offered me the job of Nephrology Director, the same title that I held at Kansas but at a university with considerably more academic clout. I was severely tempted to sign on out of respect for Dr. Robert Berliner who had left the NIH to become Dean of the Yale School of Medicine. Yale also had an extraordinarily strong Department of Physiology headed by my idol, Gerhard Giebisch. After much soul searching and discussion with Carol, I wrote to Sam to thank him for considering me and let him know that I had decided to remain at Kansas.

Word that I had looked at Yale evidently circulated among nephrology administrative circles, catching the attention of Roscoe "Ike" Robinson, M.D., the new Executive Vice-President for Health at Vanderbilt University in Nashville, Tennessee. Ike and I had met earlier in my career when he was nephrology division director at Duke and founding editor of the major academic journal in the field, "Kidney International." He had recruited me to join the executive committee of the Council on the Kidney in Cardiovascular Disease sponsored by the American Heart Association, where I met and interacted with many leaders in nephrology. I eventually became Chairman of the Council and a full member of the American Heart Association Research committee, which carried with it membership on the AHA Board of Trustees. I had plenty to do in Kansas as an NIH-supported researcher, division director, attending physician six months of every year, occasional father to my four children and absentee husband to my very busy wife. Although she didn't like it, Carol understood that opportunities for service on national committees were career-building requirements, for they increased name recognition and access to a greater cafeteria of opportunities down the road. She was confident that one day she would be included in travels to exotic places. Ike sensed that I was on an ascending career path that he wanted to pass through Vanderbilt on his watch. I had agreed to visit, fully aware that it would be hard to resist overtures from Ike Robinson, who could charm the stripes off of a zebra. I was royally hosted and toasted at lavish dinner parties and eventually offered an endowed chair to become nephrology director which, as for Yale, would be a lateral move to an institution with a stronger academic record than Kansas. I wrote detailed notes documenting the 25 interviews I had in the three days I spent on the Vanderbilt campus. At the time, Vanderbilt nephrology was in academic shambles with no one of stature to build around. There was strength in renal dialysis and transplantation, but the clinicians in those sections did not see eye to eye on several policies, meaning that the new director would have to make some Solomonic decisions the day after walking into his office. It was an opportunity to rebuild a nephrology division in an elite university with the support of the top administrative leader on the medical campus.

As I left the Vanderbilt campus, I told Ike that I was definitely interested but that I needed to meet with Carol, who knew Ike and liked him personally, and together we would think this opportunity through carefully. When I got back to the KUMC campus, I learned that word had leaked out that I was looking at Vanderbilt. Norton Greenberger, my chairman and strong backer, invited me to his office for a discussion, followed by a trip to the central administration building for an interview with the chancellor, Dr. Gene Budig. When asked why I would consider leaving Kansas, I told Dr. Budig that it was not an easy choice because KUMC was my academic home, and we were very comfortable living in Kansas. But unfortunately, the academic record of KUMC was not respected beyond Kansas and that the continued support of inept Executive Vice-Chancellors and other administrators who did not support scientific excellence worked against faculty who aspired to lift the institution to a higher academic level. He promised me, and I remember his words as clearly as the day he said them: "Jared, we need you. Stay with us, and I guarantee you that when the next EVC walks down the hall in about two years, you will be proud to shake his hand."

In the last analysis, the biggest factor that might trump the Vanderbilt opportunity was the new foundation venture with Joseph Bruening. Joe had scheduled another River Club lunch to include Ilus "Ike" Davis for a discussion of the new foundation and what our goals would be. I had said nothing to Joe about my Vanderbilt tryst, as I wanted this meeting to help me decide just what this Bruening guy was willing to do to put

PKD research on the academic map.

Ilus Davis was one of the most handsome, likeable men in the "mover and shaker class" I have ever met. Standing military-straight and more than 6 feet tall, he looked as if he had just walked out of a Hollywood casting call seeking actors to play business executives or five-star generals. He smiled widely as he shook my hand and uttered gracious words to the effect that Joe had wonderful things to say about me. I would have liked to reciprocate by stating that Joe worshiped the ground his boyhood friend walked on, but for once I kept such quips to myself.

After sitting down, we fought our way through the usual staff interruptions, then Ike took charge by abruptly asking: "Well, just what are we going to call this thing? Give me some key words."

Joe and I looked at each other, curiously, and then Joe tentatively said "Polycystic," followed haltingly by "Kidney" and "Disease."

I added "Research" and "Foundation" to the list. I think Joe added "Hope" and "Cure."

As we were lifting up these key words, Ike was writing each word on separate scraps of paper he had torn from a napkin. When we completed the list of words, Ike put them face up in the empty plate before him, looked down and studied them as he stroked his chin, then began to move the words around the plate like pieces on a chessboard. He reversed a couple of moves then proclaimed, joyously: "There, we have it! **Polycystic Kidney Research Foundation.** Now let's eat."

Joe, Ike and I enthusiastically toasted our work product for the day with raised glasses of water as I whispered, inaudibly, "This is for you, Ronnie Wilkerson."

I drove back to my office and wrote Ike Robinson a letter, graciously declining his generous offer to join him in Vanderbilt.

The PKRF was born on July 20, 1982, in the River Club on a dinner plate out of scraps of a paper napkin. We had begun what would become a thrilling journey without a map. But we had a quiver full of ideas and dreams. Joe envisioned a foundation sucking money out of the pockets of wealthy patrons, corporations and insurance companies interested in eliminating the risk of PKD. For the time being, he would rely on a small Board of Trustees including himself, his daughter Elizabeth, Ilus Davis, Ed Dillon, treasurer, and me. Joe commissioned Hal Sandy, who modernized the legendary "Smiling Jayhawk" logo of the University of Kansas athletic department and owner of a marketing business, to design the stationery and build the brand. He began to search for a part-time executive director with plans of a larger organization as funds allowed. To give the new foundation an address, he rented an inexpensive "cubby hole" office in one of his former buildings.

I was convinced that for the Foundation to be successful, we had to establish strong scientific credentials and integrity in order to persuade other researchers to join the cause. I submitted to Joe a list of candidates for a Scientific Advisory Board — the best active PKD researchers in the nation: William Bennett, M.D., University of Oregon; Kenneth Gardner, M.D., University of New Mexico; Andrew Evan, Ph.D., Indiana University; Frank Carone, M.D., Northwestern University; and myself as Chairman. Joe asked that I include Thomas Crouch, M.D. of St. Luke's Hospital, Allene Bruening's nephrologist in Kansas City. Fortunately, all agreed to serve. I don't recall who suggested the idea, but we decided that the newly-formed Scientific Advisory Board should write a Program Project Grant to the National Institutes of Health that would fund an interdisciplinary research plan. Kenneth Gardner agreed to serve as Program Director. If we could land the first multi-institutional research grant to explore the biology and pathology of renal cystic disease, it would give the new Foundation instant credibility among renal scientists and clinicians.

CHAPTER 26

Building critical mass

With the creation of the PKRF, we stepped up the pace to find a treatment for PKD. Joe Bruening asked again how long I thought it would take to get there. My reply this time went beyond promising our best effort. I asked if he had ever heard of "Sutton's Law of medical research" and he had not, nor did he know that Willie Sutton was a notorious bank robber.

"When Willie was finally caught," I explained, "a captor asked him, 'Willie, why do you rob banks?' To which Willie replied, 'Because that's where the money is.'"

"I get it, Jared. I've got to raise lots of cash to attract the scientist bank robbers to take money for PKD research."

The journey began when Joseph Bruening set up an impressive PKD bank that looked like money, but which in fact only had Joe's checkbook in the vault. History will show that it took several hundred scientists 30 years and hundreds of millions of dollars of private and federal loot before the first treatment specifically targeting PKD was announced in 2012.

Hal Sandy, who spells his name $andy in private correspondence, was commissioned to design stationery and information brochures that "looked like money." Joe recruited Jean Bacon as a part-time Executive

Director of the PKRF as well as one part-time administrative assistant who occupied a tiny office outfitted with scruffy furnishings, a telephone and antiquated equipment.

I contacted James Scherbenske, Ph.D., a former fellow in Larry Sullivan's lab at KUMC, who was the administrator for most of the kidney physiology grants funded by the Kidney Urology and Hematology Section at the National Institutes of Health. I explained that we had gathered a group of "cyst watchers" (Gardner referred to us as "The Brotherhood of Cysters") to formulate a Program Project Grant on PKD with a multi-center basis. Sherbenske took the idea to Nancy Cummings, M.D., head of the Kidney Urology Hematology Section, who liked it and recommended that we go ahead with the submission. Scherbenske was assigned to oversee the scientific peer review. Joe pledged his financial support making it possible for those of us in the group to meet face-to-face to discuss and critique the draft components of the proposal. Larry and Dan Welling from KUMC joined Ken Gardner, William Bennett, Andrew Evan and Frank Carone from our newly-formed Scientific Advisory Committee of the PKRF to write the Program Project Grant. Gardner submitted the $1,400,000 request from the University of New Mexico in 1983.

Joe frantically wrote letters on the new stationery to every wealthy person he knew, pleading for money to support this worthy new venture. A few replies came back with relatively small amounts of money; nonetheless, he was relentless in making contacts and following through. He turned up a saint when Gordon Flesch, CEO of the Gordon Flesch Company in Madison, Wisconsin, answered his call and signed on as a new member of the Board of Trustees. Adding this perfect gentleman to the BOT was a huge lift for Joe, and it was fun seeing this distraught man come alive and display newfound energy and clever wit. His verve spilled over into the quasi-science area, and almost daily, I would receive a letter from him, together with a newspaper article or magazine story about a new diet or treatment for kidney disease that more often than not had no scientific basis. Once, when I dashed the importance of rutabagas in health, Joe said, a little perturbed at my intransigence, "Now Jared, if some scientist believed that eating almonds would make you feel better, would there be any harm if I ate a lot of almonds to find out if they helped?"

I replied that it would help the almond farmer make a profit, but without having a scientific analysis to back up the claim of benefit, I thought that almond therapy would fall into the snake-oil catalog of nostrums sold to those who are desperately uncritical. I used this almond issue to introduce him to placebo effects and to explain how scientists design crucial experiments in humans to avoid bias by not letting the patient or the administering physician know who is actually getting the new medication.

I thought he had really flipped when he paid for a small, but very expensive advertisement in the Wall Street Journal seeking persons to join him in his worthy cause fighting polycystic disease. It ran only once and netted a CEO from Oklahoma City, John Gammill, who signed on and matched Joe's generosity for many years. (Former KUMC faculty member Benjamin Cowley, M.D. now holds the John Gammill Chair in Polycystic Kidney Disease at the University of Oklahoma.)

Allene was stricken with a life-threatening blood infection that probably originated in a kidney cyst. Antibiotics given by vein suppressed the infection, but as soon as they were discontinued, it would flare up again. Fortunately, I was in position to help out. A year earlier, I had persuaded a resident in Internal Medicine, Steven Schwab M.D., to collect cyst fluids from the nephrectomy specimen of a patient with unrelenting renal infections who had failed treatment with a host of different antibiotics. With the help of Dan Hinthorn, M.D. in the Infectious Diseases Division and Dennis Diederich, M.D. in Nephrology, he measured antibiotic levels and pH in the fluids of several cysts. Although clindamycin is not a good drug for the type of bacteria usually found in kidney infections, we had used it in this case in desperation to cover all potential organisms. Once again, chance was on our side, for when the data finally came in, we found that the concentrations of clindamycin were very high in cysts that registered high acid levels, i.e. low pH. Further analysis indicated that clindamycin was accumulating within cysts similar to the way that ammonia, a strong base, accumulates in the urine.

We knew on the basis of long-standing basic renal physiology studies that ammonia is normally trapped in the urine of collecting ducts before it flows into the urinary bladder to be discharged. We reasoned that the chemical properties of clindamycin caused it to be trapped in acid urine as well. It was reasonable to suppose that cysts containing acid pH fluids would accumulate high levels of drugs with chemical properties similar to clindamycin. Before it was published, I discussed our data with Bill Bennett, a member of the new Scientific Advisory Board of the PKRF. Bill decided to look for antibiotics with the same properties as clindamycin, but with a better profile for killing bacteria in the urinary tract. To get the ball rolling for Mrs. Bruening, I asked Bennett to submit to the PKRF the grant proposal he had planned to send as part of our PPG. The scientific advisory committee, absent Bill Bennett, reviewed and approved the grant.

I presented our antibiotic distribution data at a meeting of nephrologists in Milan, Italy, and challenged the audience to help us find something with a wider spectrum than clindamycin. Thinking that my challenge would go unheeded, I headed for my seat only to be called back to the podium by the moderator to take a comment from the floor. Eberhard Ritz, M.D. from Heidelberg had raised his hand and stood to speak.

At the time, Ritz was an up-start nephrologist on the world stage. Fluent in five languages and exceedingly bright and well read, he struck fear into the hearts of more poorly prepared physicians with whom he sought to duel.

"Professor, Grantham," I can still hear his authoritative tone, "If you lived in a more advanced part of the world, you would already know that Bayer (a German pharmaceutical company) has a gyrase inhibitor in clinical trials that fits your requirements perfectly."

This was news to me — good news — and I dismissed his patrician manner to thank him for the tip and for bringing this constructive information to my attention. When the session ended, we sought each other out and proceeded to have a civil discussion during which he praised me for using fundamental physiology to solve clinical problems, and I complimented him for knowing the chemical properties of a drug that was not yet on the market.

Carol accompanied me on the trip to Milan, a small reward for being left alone with the children while I was building a career and thinking about urine. The program organizer had arranged to take some of the invited speakers and their wives to the opening of the opera season at La Scala featuring Placido Domingo and Shirley Verette in "Carmen." An intestinal virus hit Carol, who had spent two days visiting the sights of Milan while I was in meetings, within a few hours of the scheduled opera. We are both opera buffs and a chance to attend opening night at La Scala was a once in a lifetime opportunity. Nothing deters this woman when she has set her mind to do something, so she bundled up and we pushed off to La Scala. About 10 of us in the party had to "share" a booth on the third floor at the back of the stunningly beautiful, iconic auditorium. There were two chairs at the front, one of which Carol sat in. I stood with the men through the opera, supremely happy just to be there, but more respectful of sardines, once the opera ended.

Princess Caroline of Monaco had walked by us in the foyer and was seated at the front of the box directly below Carol. I cautioned my bride that it would be most unseemly were she to vomit on the Princess during the opera. Fortunately, Carol kept her intestines in check, and she ate sparingly as we dined late into the night after the performance. Around 3 am, we were awakened by a telephone call with the news that all Italian airports were closed due to a strike. A bus had been ordered that would take us to Zurich where we would get on an airplane to Washington, D.C. Several other speakers in Milan and I were scheduled to give talks at the Annual Meeting of the American Society of Nephrology (ASN) the following day. It was an interesting moonlit ride through the Italian and Swiss Alps. Gary Striker, M.D. and his wife, Liliane, were on the bus with us. Our incarceration together for several hours on the bus and in transit to Washington made it easy to get better acquainted — and was my good fortune. Gary had just been named the new Director of the Kidney Urology and Hematology Division of the NIDDK in the National Institutes of Health.

I cornered Bill Bennett at the ASN meeting and told him of Ritz's comment about the Bayer drug. Bill took charge and literally smuggled some of the pills into the United States, which Allene Bruening received by mouth and was cured. The new antibiotic turned out to be Ciprofloxacin. It and drugs like it have become the "Gold Standard" agents for treating complex renal infections in PKD patients. I think this story illustrates nicely that basic and clinical scientists working together toward a goal of treating a particular disease have enormously greater discovery power than if they toil separately in research silos. Another irony in this tale: The first grant funded by the PKRF proved to be profoundly helpful to the founder's wife. And it was gratifying to experience first-hand that this conservative businessman understood that he had received an amazing early return on his investment.

Adding to that success was the exciting news in 1984 that our Program Project Grant would be funded by the NIH, validating the PKRF vision that we were in the business to encourage that high quality science be brought to bear to understand the cause and find treatments and a cure for PKD. We extended our reach to the scientific community and practicing physicians in 1984 by holding a meeting in Kansas City, Missouri, on the theme "Problems in diagnosis and management of polycystic disease." We invited 22 international scientists and clinicians to meet for two days and discuss all aspects of PKD. The presentations and the discussions that followed were transcribed and published in book-form by Hal Sandy in an elegant collection that established the PKRF and the researchers in this field of study as a force to be taken seriously. Perhaps the most significant benefit that derived from the actual meeting was that Vicente Torres, M.D., a participant from the Mayo Clinic, was so impressed with the activities of the PKRF that he decided to turn a major portion of his research program toward PKD.

In 1983, newspapers had announced that the chromosomal location of the mutated gene causing Huntington's Chorea had been located, a major step forward toward nailing down the cause of the condition that took the life of Woody Guthrie. Huntington's is a degenerative brain condition inherited in an autosomal dominant pattern like PKD, meaning that each child of an affected parent has a 50/50 chance of inheriting the gene defect. To localize the Huntington's gene, a new strategy called *linkage analysis* had been utilized. Autosomal dominant PKD (ADPKD) is much more prevalent than Huntington's, so the news inspired members of the PKRF scientific advisory committee to petition the NIDDK to fund studies to look for the location of the ADPKD gene.

Letters were exchanged, and after several months, several other advisors and I travelled to the NIH to meet with Dr. Gary Striker, director of the Kidney Urology and Hematology section of the NIDDK. Before he joined the NIH, Dr. Striker had established a strong investigative record at the University of Washington. He had also studied polycystic kidney disease and proved to be a strong ally. We made our case for issuing a request for proposals (RFP) to do linkage studies in PKD families knowing that if we could localize then clone the gene, we would have the cause of the disease in hand.

In one sense, single gene disorders, like infectious diseases, are easier to study than more complex, acquired maladies like diabetes, lupus and cancer because the cause resides in defective (mutated) DNA that is passed from parent to child. Find the mutated gene and you have the cause and can work toward understanding how the abnormality causes disease mayhem. Since we did not have a candidate gene to work from in our new Program Project studies, we had to look at what the disease had done to the kidneys and work back to figure out what might be causing the damage.

I think the approach we took to finding a cure for PKD is analogous to building the first trans-continental railroad: One construction team began on the Pacific side of the continent and labored over high mountains and deserts toward the east while the Atlantic team whizzed westward on relatively flat land. The separate teams finally met at Provo, Utah, where the golden spike was driven in to signify that the tracks uniting the nation were completely aligned. By analogy, those of us on the Program Project team started on the "Pacific" side and moved east at a snail's pace, turning up kernels of new knowledge that could be patched together to prove that cysts grew endlessly because they were driven to abnormal growth and fluid accumulation by the hormone vasopressin (anti-diuretic hormone). We were anxious for the day when the new tools of molecular biology and gene manipulation would be available so the team on the "Atlantic" side could ignite a streamlined dash heading west to determine the molecular cause of PKD.

Before the ink had dried on the NIH request for proposals to localize the PKD gene, word reached the PKRF in 1985 that Stephen Reeders, M.D., a research fellow working alone in the laboratory of a famous hematologist at Oxford, had localized a PKD gene on chromosome 16 in several large families in England and the Netherlands. The paper was scheduled to be published in "Nature." The infant PKRF staff wondered why that public announcement could not be made in Kansas City on the campus of the Kansas University Medical Center. On behalf of the PKRF, I contacted Reeders and asked if he would be willing to come to Kansas City to give a lecture and make the announcement at a press conference the same day the paper was scheduled to be published. He said he was game, and so we welcomed the youthful scientist to the KUMC campus where he delivered his talk with the aplomb of a seasoned professional.

Prior to the lecture, the PKRF office had notified Cable News Network of the talk, which they kindly reported as a public service announcement mentioned during several national newscasts. Bryce Reynolds, a mortgage broker in California, happened to catch the CNN broadcast and contacted the PKRF office to see if he and his wife, Lova, would be permitted to attend Reeders' lecture. Indeed, they were welcome! They flew to Kansas City, met with Reeders after his talk, and later pledged money to the PKRF in support of Reeders' future research to isolate and characterize the miscreant gene. It was a whirlwind meeting sandwiched between my clinical and administrative responsibilities, but I learned once more that the slightest national advertising can yield excellent results when it is properly targeted. Bryce later became chairman of the Board of Trustees of the PKRF, and Reeders was ultimately persuaded to take a faculty position at Yale in the Howard Hughes Institute.

Suddenly, PKD research gained the attention of renal and other scientists who sensed that the cause of the disorder would soon be deciphered from the genetic code in the chunk of DNA containing the mistaken molecule. However, things got more complex when William Kimberling, Ph.D. working with Patricia Gabow, M.D. and Robert Schrier, M.D. at the University of Colorado discovered another chromosomal DNA site. We now had to deal with PKD1 and PKD2. In research, complexity is the grist of discovery and new knowledge. The National Institutes of Health, with the internal support of Gary Striker, rose to the occasion by declaring that proposals for PKD research would receive priority consideration. This and effective liaison with select members of the federal House and Senate committees on health mediated by Warren Elliott, the PKRF's "Washington representative," provided the resources to support new grants from the NIH. At last, PKD research had broken out of Dangerfield's doldrums and was getting deserved attention.

Meanwhile, as a member of the Program Project Grant led by Ken Gardner, I was having success redefining the pathology of discarded cystic kidneys removed from patients in preparation for renal transplantation. I decided to momentarily put aside the search for a chemical that caused fluid to be pumped into the cysts thinking that we needed a better understanding of just what a cyst was. I had collected and preserved several worn-out polycystic kidneys and enlisted research assistant James Geiser to examine hundreds of cysts by high-powered scanning electron microscopy with the goal of describing the micro-anatomy of cysts from the time they developed within a kidney tubule the size of a human hair up to the point they were 2 to 3 inches in diameter. This project was analogous to describing the Grand Canyon by traipsing around it taking pictures of interesting rock formations. However, our simple study had scientific payoffs far greater than I ever expected, for it helped to prove that individual cysts were products of excessive cell proliferation; that cysts were lined by a single layer of epithelial cells; and moreover, that about three-quarters of the cysts had completely separated from the tubules in which they had formed. Finding that most of the cysts were isolated sacs of fluid with no outlets meant that the only way the fluid within them could increase was by being actively secreted through the cellular walls into the lumen. It seemed that I could not escape the "fluid secretion" muse, so I began to think once again about how liquid might be secreted into the cysts.

Perhaps the cysts had borrowed molecular mechanisms from tear ducts, sweat glands and the small intestine, tissues known to generate fluid products represented by tears, perspiration and watery diarrhea. Were that to be the case, I would still be bound to attack the nephrology canon proscribing that "kidneys only filter and reabsorb fluid." To prove that they could secrete fluid would require more than the anatomic data I had in hand.

A way to address my secretion hypothesis came in a momentous demonstration by James McAteer, Ph.D. and Andrew Evan, Ph.D. at a regularly scheduled meeting of our new PKD Program Project group in 1985. These investigators had learned through word of mouth that Patricia Wilson, Ph.D., in the new PKD center at the University of Colorado, had successfully grown cyst epithelial cells from the walls of discarded human kidneys in synthetic medium. McAteer and Evan had recently confirmed Wilson's breakthrough method and showed our Program Project team, in gorgeous photo-micrographs and time-lapse photographs, proof that epithelial cells lining the internal surfaces of transected human cysts literally "walked out of the cyst" and grew onto the plastic surface of a culture dish. They also demonstrated that when immortalized kidney epithelial cells derived from a dog's kidney (Madin Darby Canine Kidney, MDCK cells) were suspended within a Jello-like matrix, they continued to reproduce and form tiny fluid-filled cysts that enlarged day after day. These findings meant that we now had ways to examine specific growth and functional properties of the actual cells that make up human cysts in a highly controlled environment outside of the human body. Thanks to these advances, I now had the means to definitively test the hypothesis that renal cyst epithelial cells secrete fluid and, thereby, contribute to the overall renal enlargement process that is the hallmark of PKD.

However, I was not trained in cell culture methods nor was anyone in our Nephrology group at the University of Kansas. I was due for another sabbatical leave, so I discussed the possibility with Carol that we return to the NIH where I could learn cell culture methods and molecular biology from my old friends, Moe Burg and Joseph Handler, who had recently adopted cell culture to investigate renal cell biology.

All of our children were out of the house. Janeane had graduated from Baker University and had earned her BSN degree at the University of Kansas. A staff nurse working in the KU Hospital, she met and married Jerry Houchin, a respiratory therapist in the hospital. They were expecting our first grandchild. Jared Taylor graduated from Baker with a degree in business and psychology and had married Julie Earnshaw before the start of their junior year. Taylor was the owner of Taylor Lawn and Landscape located in Overland Park, Kansas. James Aaron was a senior in pre-medical studies at the University of Kansas and Joel Don, a sophomore at KU, was majoring in aeronautical engineering. Our only family concern was my father, Jimmie, who in retirement had developed diabetes mellitus and was losing weight. He had tried and failed to lose weight all of his life, and now it was falling off without any effort.

Carol and I thought carefully and decided that it would be a good time for me to wind down a bit, even if it meant being away from our first grandchild. One additional benefit of studying in Bethesda was that my sister, Annetta, lived in Silver Spring, Maryland, with her husband, Jay Batchelder, and daughters, Jenna and Jessica. Annie was the head nurse of the labor and delivery deck at the Bethesda Naval Hospital, located across Rockville Pike from the National Institutes of Health where I would be working. I called Moe Burg to see if he had room for me, and he accepted my proposal on the spot. I met with my chairman at KUMC, and together we petitioned the Dean of Medicine for a nine-month leave for educational enhancement that began in the fall of 1986.

After decades of beauty shop wear and tear, one of my mother's hip joints had worn out and was causing excruciating pain. I made arrangements for her surgery and rehabilitation at the KU Hospital before we were scheduled to begin the sabbatical leave in September. There was a humorous moment in the hospital waiting room on the day her operation was scheduled. Carol and my father were anxiously waiting for a report from the operating room on my mother's condition. A woman clothed in surgical attire popped into the room and asked if any members of the Grantham family were present. My father leaped to his feet, but his pants did not come with him, and for a few seconds, he stood before 20 or 30 onlookers in only his boxer underwear. Carol helped him to regain his composure, pulled up his pants and fastened them tightly so they could find out what the messenger had to say. It turns out she had only an interim report that Mrs. Grantham was doing just fine and the surgery should be completed within an hour. We were all together later when the surgeon reported on his handiwork, after which we had a good laugh, acknowledging that my father, the village clown, had stolen the show again. I was so preoccupied with Mother's surgery and our impending escape to Bethesda that it did not occur to me that his weight loss was a harbinger of trouble ahead.

Ashley Laine Houchin was born shortly before we were to leave, an event Carol and I had been looking forward to, although we would be denied opportunities to over-cuddle her while we were in Maryland. Jerry and Janeane moved into our house, saving them some money while housesitting. Moe and Joe found us a furnished townhouse a block south of the NIH campus. I could walk to the lab through the massive green campus studded with huge trees and flowering bushes leaving Carol with the car for her diverse journeys during the day. We settled in for what we thought would be another bucolic sabbatical and more quality time together.

I had lost status since I left the Laboratory of Kidney and Electrolyte Metabolism in 1969. I was assigned to a desk in a room shared with six renal fellows, most of who had just begun to shave. I dressed down to match their attire and dug into the job at hand, learning to culture renal cells without contaminating the entire NIH. Joe had a small project he wanted me to do, so I got up to speed and began to get some results we could believe. Sadly, the experiment failed, but not because of me. In research, failure happens more often than success — you just don't read about the negative results in the science journals.

Before we knew it, Christmas was upon us, and we returned to Kansas City to be with our family. We squeezed into the house along with Janeane, Jerry and Ashley, even managing to find room for my parents. Uncle Taylor, Uncle Aaron and Uncle Joel had their pictures taken holding their first niece. At the gift exchange, Aaron and Joel, now fraternity brothers at KU, exchanged checks for $200, each emoting that they didn't know how much the other cared.

My father pulled me aside to report that he had been having sharp pains "over his plate" as he pointed to his pubic area. I quizzed him over and over about the discomfort but couldn't be sure what the "plate" was and whether it was serious or just bowel gas. I did a cursory examination of his abdomen, this time noting his weight loss. I couldn't feel any lumps or elicit the pain he complained about. We were scheduled to return to Bethesda shortly, so I asked him to contact his doctor at home about the pain if it persisted or got worse and let me know if they found anything.

While at home, I checked in with my nephrology colleagues at KUMC and learned that they were very busy but had kept everything glued together. The senior research assistants in my laboratory were making excellent progress on various projects. The PKRF was also doing fine without me around. So we headed back to Bethesda to continue my science upgrade.

❖

CHAPTER 27

More shaping

In February, my father's abdominal pain got so bad that his family physician sent him to Garden City, Kansas, to have a colonoscopy. The gastroenterologist reported that he saw a mass projecting into the left descending colon, but he chose not to biopsy it. I decided that we must return to Kansas City and admit my father to the KU Hospital for a complete evaluation. Friends in Johnson City brought my parents to our home in Overland Park where I met them. My father, in considerable discomfort, was admitted to the General Internal Medicine Service, given pain relief and a repeat colonoscopy scheduled for the following morning.

The gastroenterologist, an old hand at this kind of thing, was certain that my father had an adenocarcinoma in his descending colon. No one could come up with an alternative explanation for his lower abdominal pain that had been there since late summer. One of the outstanding surgeons at the KU Hospital, who did kidney transplants for us in the early years, was called to do an operation. My father was taken to surgery, and I took my mother and Carol to the nephrology office to await the news. I told the surgeon he could find us in the nephrology library. In less than two hours, he walked into the library grim-faced. He explained, obviously a little shaken by his findings, that my father had widespread pancreatic cancer in his abdomen. The colon tumor was in fact an inva-sive pancreatic cancer and the pain in the lower abdomen was caused by the invasion of tumor cells. Unfortunately, there was nothing he could do except close him up tight.

In a case like this, chemotherapy was out of the question, leaving only palliative care. In recovery, my father suffered massive clotting of his left femoral vein requiring the use of anticoagulants. Amazingly, the clot cleared in a few days, and he was judged stable enough to take home to Johnson, the place he longed to go. I bought a small van in which we fashioned a bed he could lie on during the 450-mile journey across Kansas. He did amazingly well, requiring only small amounts of analge-sics. He called out the different villages and places of interest he and my mother had driven past on their many trips to Kansas City to be with us. He had a story to tell about each one. Naturally, they knew all the good eating places having run their own restaurant in Johnson for 10 years.

His family physician was there to greet us as we pulled into the am-bulance entrance at the hospital in Johnson City. He assured me that they would take good care of my father and would not let him suffer. This from the man who told me during one of my visits to just say hello when I was in Johnson visiting family, "You know, Jared, it takes three minutes to write a valium prescription; 30 minutes not to." It was com-forting to know that this man understood the proper use of narcotics and tranquilizers.

Johnson City rallied once again for the Grantham family, sending em-issaries to visit my father on a regular basis. His half-brother, Dennis Hall, the good-hearted uncle my sons and I had idolized in youth, planned to stay in Johnson and help my mother manage. An alumnus of the pickle barrel brouhaha and other family squabbles, this was a way to diminish a long-standing debt he believed he owed to his brother. With so many saints looking after him, Carol and I seized the opportunity to return to Bethesda to take care of unfinished business left in our hasty exit.

Moe and Joe were very gracious about my absences, explaining that they didn't really expect much productivity from me in the first place and to just relax and take in as much technology and new science as I could manage. I had begun to formulate new experiments related to polycystic kidney disease that I wanted to do upon returning full-time to Kansas.

News from Johnson was not good. My father found it difficult to eat solid or liquid food and was rapidly losing weight. We made plans to return to Johnson City in a week. During the evening of March 27, 1987, Carol and I saw a Woody Allen movie, "Radio Days," in the Bethesda Theater on Rockville Pike, then went home and turned in. Around 3 am, the telephone rang and it was Aaron on the line trying hard to speak over his sobbing cry. We had been expecting a call about my father. I wondered why Aaron was calling and not Uncle Dennis.

"It's Joel, Dad. He's dead."

I had trouble understanding him and didn't want to hear what I thought he'd said.

"Okay, Aaron. Try again to tell me what you just said."

"Joel was hit by a train. In a car with three other friends," he managed to say more clearly.

I don't remember the details of the conversation that followed except that Aaron was crying uncontrollably and I felt as though all of my blood had suddenly disappeared. After several false starts, we managed to get the conversation moving again, and Aaron handed the phone to a State Patrolman, who had brought the devastating news to our house in Overland Park and was waiting to speak to me.

Carol had overheard everything and was weeping uncontrollably. We embraced each other as tears flowed in surges. I found it difficult to bring the phone to my ear. The officer, who waited for me to respond, was calm and professional, evidently having been given the task of speaking to grieving parents many times in the past. He explained that our son had been riding in a car owned by Joel's best friend and fraternity brother, Dan McDevitt, along with college friends Elizabeth Dunlap and Jennifer Jones. They were all killed instantly when the car was struck by a fast-moving freight train as they drove across an unguarded crossing north of Lawrence.

"Did you find his wallet?"

"Yes. His driver's license picture matches."

"Does he have blond hair?"

"Yes."

With no more room to bargain for mistaken identity, I thanked the officer saying that we would be coming back to Kansas City in a few hours and would contact the morgue about what to do with Joel's remains.

I called Braniff Airlines and booked two seats on a direct flight to Kansas City leaving at 8 am that morning, then called Aaron to let him know when we would be arriving in Kansas City. Janeane, Taylor and Aaron met us at the exit gate in the airport. I collapsed in Taylor's arms and Carol in Aaron's. We managed to gather our luggage and drive to our home for a tearful reunion with Jerry and Ashley. Later in the day, Taylor, Aaron and I drove to Lawrence to inspect the site of the accident and to gather Joel's things at the fraternity house.

I am embarrassed to admit that I cannot recall how Carol handled much of this. I had been able to compartmentalize stressful events and situations in my medical practice and still be sensitive to the needs of others; however, in this un-Godly crucible, the emotional pain penetrated so deep that my knees buckled each time a relative or friend would embrace me. At times, I seemed to be operating in a parallel universe, struggling feebly to maintain some degree of equanimity.

Carol had called my sister, Annetta, before we left Bethesda for the airport. After an emotional meltdown, Annie said she would join us in Kansas City as soon as she could arrange her affairs. Our second day in Kansas City was filled by well-wishers coming to leave food and visits by teams of professionals representing insurance agencies that covered the wrecked automobile and the Union Pacific Railroad. The automobile insurance adjustor got there first and explained the kind of financial help we could expect from his company. He did offer his opinion that Union Pacific had created a distraction by parking a train a few yards to the right of the crossing with a bright headlight turned on. He was convinced that a driver approaching the unguarded crossing would focus on the parked train and be distracted because there was no brakeman on the ground to tell him if it was safe to pass in front of the engine. A fast-moving train coming from the left hit the car.

The railroad representatives came next and expressed their condolences and sorrow and assured us that the engineer was emotionally shaken by the encounter because his effort to stop the train came to no avail. I was anxious to get everyone who was not friend or family out of the house and kept both meetings short and to the point. The lives of four precious young students on the threshold of adulthood were wiped out in an instant and money or gratuitous words would not bring them back.

Our minister came by in the afternoon, and we discussed the elements of a memorial service. I have an aversion to viewing dead loved ones, as my creepy brain stores that as the person's last image, a vision that is recalled whenever the deceased's name is lifted up. Carol and I agreed that the casket would not be present at the service; those in the family who had to see Joel to gain closure would have that opportunity the evening before at a viewing to be held at the mortuary. My surviving memory of Joel recalls an effervescent young man surging into the house through the front door yelling "Hi" to whoever was around before he attacked the fridge and took a quick drink out of the orange juice bottle.

On the flight from Washington to Kansas City, I had penned some words that Carol and I wanted to be used in Joel's memorial service at our church in Overland Park. "Joel Don Grantham: In memorium" was read by Mr. Leslie Holdeman on March 30, 1987.

> The birth in Bethesda, Maryland, of a third son, the fourth child, brightened the cold January days of 1967 for Carol and Jared. Joel Grantham's arrival, though routine and unheralded, would be special in so many ways. This would be the last child for the young couple from the Midwest.

His first and middle names were retrieved from Jared's past — two young men whose lives were stilled by polio in youth's bud. Joel would memorialize their names in tribute to courage, and dreams unfulfilled. He honored their names in his own being, for if there was ever a child, a son, a brother, an uncle or a grandson who was perfect, Joel personified the description.

Joel was a member of the Grantham fairy kingdom under the reign of Princess Janeane. Taylor the Toad, Aaron the Worm and Joel the Mole would live their own "Wind-in-the-willows" saga in the years to come — brothers looking out for one another under the loving scrutiny and guidance of an older sister.

Growing up brought opportunities for community participation. Joel was baptized in the Methodist Church and prepared for service in the Indian Heights family. He was "White Lightening" in the YMCA Indian Guides, paired with his father, "Big Thunder," and later a WEBELOS, Cub and Boy Scout.

In the early years of Commanche Elementary School, Joel was the shortest, but also the fastest lad in his class. Two towering older brothers soon raised the issue of height to a sensitive level, and Joel, with the adoring assistance of Grandpa Grantham, would record in indelible ink his progress toward manhood on a wall in the garage. Over some intervals of time when progress was slow, we think Grandpa may have "fudged" the marks a centimeter or two to raise his grandson's spirits.

Size did not prevent Joel from participating in basketball, football and baseball in elementary and junior high school. In senior high, he endured the tortures of competitive wrestling, but golf was really his favorite game. He learned to play the trumpet and became a member of the Shawnee Mission High School marching and jazz bands. An occasional few bars of a trumpet solo were kind rewards for hard work and unswerving devotion to his band and to his school.

He studied hard, earned recognition as a member of the National Honor Society and received a scholarship to study aeronautical engineering at the University of Kansas. He was initiated into the Phi Gamma Delta social fraternity and served as the Scholarship Chairman in the sophomore year. He loved his fraternity brothers, and he was loved by them. That's the kind of guy Joel was, dependable, unassuming, quietly caring — not much for flash or fury, but a steady constructive force in his family and his community.

When life ends in youth, one hasn't time to mark the shortened path with monuments of stone or words. The memorials are the poignant images carried in the hearts and minds of those who knew and loved Joel. Remembrances that will never let us forget him, remembrances such as these that will soften the pain of his loss with the joy of his life:

"Hi, Mom. I'm home!"

"Guess what, Joel?"

"What, Dad?"

"I'm not as hungry as I used to be."

"Hi, Neenie!"

"Yoel Grinner."

"Move over, Chewy!"

In his senior year of high school, Joel was troubled, as many young people are, by the suffocating realization of his own mortality. He and his father talked through his concerns and, as so typified this man, he fought this fear and conquered it. At Christmas time 1986, he calmly reported to both parents, "You know, I'm not afraid of dying anymore."

Joel Don Grantham was born on January 10, 1967. He was in love with life, right up to the end, in the night of March 27, 1987.

And he was not afraid.

Mike and Diane Linshaw, dear friends who had watched our children grow up, flew back from their home in Connecticut to attend Joel's memorial service. During the reception that followed, Mike and I discussed the imminent death of my father and how the family should deal with my mother who would be alone 450 miles from the nearest close relative. Mike had worked through this problem with his mother and advised that we let my mom decide what she wanted to do. He predicted — or better, prophesized — that she would want to stay in her home in a community that knew and cared for her.

My sister, Annetta, and her family had driven from Silver Spring to attend Joel's service and had moved on to visit our parents in Johnson City, neither of whom could attend Joel's service. On April 1st, Annie called to tell us that my father had died peacefully and that she was at his side. Cut from the same cloth as her father, she also averred, "Wasn't it just like that guy to check out on April Fool's Day." Arrangements were being made to have his service in two days. She took care of notifying relatives knowing that we were still struggling to adjust to our other crushing loss.

We gathered our children and caravanned to Johnson City to celebrate the life of "The kindest man in Stanton County," the title of the second eulogy I wrote to assuage grief in the winter of 1987. The church was packed with well-wishers. In a tribute to our father's frequent clownish enthusiasm, Annie purchased multi-colored helium-filled balloons that were released at the conclusion of the graveside burial service.

While in Johnson City, I managed to get in a quick visit to meet with Ronnie Wilkerson, who happened to be on dialysis in his home.

After three failed attempts at renal transplantation in the University of Colorado program, he was terribly discouraged. Talking with him helped me to refocus my grief into more constructive work that needed to be done more urgently. On the return to Kansas City, I stopped by my lab and laid out the new approach we would soon be taking to study polycystic kidney disease using the methods I had learned and modified during the sabbatical. We eventually made it back to Bethesda where my friends in the Laboratory of Kidney and Electrolyte Metabolism warmly received me.

As Mike Linshaw had predicted, my brave mother decided to remain in Johnson. Uncle Dennis, to his saintly credit, stayed long enough to help her get adjusted to living alone. Carol and I found it difficult to generate any excitement about remaining in Bethesda. We did things, saw things and travelled about, but there was little joy in any of it. I did discover the minicomputer and bought an Apple Macintosh. I had found the IBM DOS language intimidating, but the intuitive Mac changed that. I worked on expository writing, syntax and developing a writing style. I discovered that preoccupation with sentence composition and structure would drive the harsher memories and intrusive thoughts out of my head.

One beautiful Saturday afternoon in May, Carol and I walked over to the NIH campus to just sit on the grass, read and enjoy the warm breezes. There was enchantment in the air as the 17-year cicadas were singing furiously for their mates and the high-pitched sound wafted over us, occasionally in great rushes. I had a yellow pad to jot down any new research ideas that might seep into my consciousness; instead, a strange calmness came over me I had never experienced before, and I was compelled to write verse about Mount Oread, the hill that Kansas University is built on and that Carol and I had lived on the first year of our marriage. The words came to me as though they had been transcribed previously:

Spirit of Mount Oread

A glacial mound,
Some rain and wind,
One million years,
or two, or ten.
Til on its crown,
Proud University,
Towers o'er the Kaw
Through all eternity.

Ten thousand souls
Have walked the hill.
A century
That could not still
The love of friends,
Who share as one,
The Spirit's sound
In the carillion.

Who can explain,
Who could foretell,
The new dimension
On that hill?
It calls a lassie,
And a lad.
Come, find the Spirit
Of Oread.

Outrageous youth
Of flesh and sin.
A task to mold,
A chance to win
The race against
Frivolity,
To taste the fruit
Of Society.

So much to have,
And more to give.
Against such odds,
Oh, let them live
To spread their seed,
To futures add,
And magnify
The Spirit of Oread.

If life should end,
Before they've trod,
On down the hill,
Received the nod,
Will they belong
Among the best?
Will memories fade,
As their souls rest?

"Do not despair,
Your child is here.
We are at peace,
We know no fear.
We will enjoy
Eternal youth
Upon this hill,
That is the truth."

Spirit of Life!
Spirit of Truth!
Spirit of Love!
Spirit of Youth!
Oh, blessed hill,
Our hearts can see,
The sweet communion of this place,
Through all eternity.

It was as though our child and his friends were transmitting from that hill the words I heard and wrote down — words that helped to temper the searing pain of grief. The poem was eventually printed in the University of Kansas student newspaper, The Daily Kansan. Carol and I commissioned John Pozdro, Professor of Composition at Kansas University, to write a musical setting for mixed voices and organ. An elite choir performed "Spirit of Mount Oread" on November 4, 1990, in a memorial concert on the KU campus.

❖

CHAPTER 28

When vision partners with intuition

The first experiment I did upon returning to KUMC was to duplicate the new culture technique McAteer and Evan had worked out with the dog kidney line of immortalized cells called MDCK. When the individual cells were embedded in a Jello-like matrix and "fed" with a liquid resembling blood plasma, little cysts formed and grew indefinitely. When they got large enough, they looked like gas bubbles in the translucent Jello-like mold that supported their growth. In this way, we could grow as many cysts as we needed to answer key questions about PKD.

This crucial technical advance also helped me to realize, in an "Ah Ha! moment," that renal cysts were in fact the simplest three dimensional, multi-cellular structures in human biology — a single, continuous layer of cells capable of secreting fluid. Think of cysts as water-filled balloons in which the fluid is constrained by the thin layer of rubber representing the *epithelial* wall. In a balloon, the liquid is pushed in through a single hole, whereas in the cysts the fluid it literally pumped in through millions of microscopic holes called *pores* that penetrate the epithelial cells. Obviously, the most important physiologic processes needed to form cysts that progressively enlarge are: one, reproduction of the cells (*proliferation*) making up the wall of the cyst so that it can expand, and two, secretion of fluid into the potential cavity generated by the expanding cyst wall.

The discovery of a process with such obvious components is perhaps more aptly labeled a "Duh moment." But that is how research works. Not infrequently, the obvious is overlooked. When McAteer and Evan reduced the process of cyst formation and growth down to the simplest model, research questions began to fly out of my head like fleas off my dog Toby.

Before the faculty of medicine at KUMC, I pointed out the similarities between the growth of malignant cancers and renal cysts. Kurt Ebner, Ph.D., Chairman of Biochemistry, came up to me after the lecture to tell me that he was intrigued by the relationships between PKD and neoplastic growth (*neoplasia = neoplastic = new growth*) and suggested that I get together with James Calvet, Ph.D. to discuss a collaboration. Calvet was the first molecular biologist recruited to the KU faculty in the Department of Biochemistry, meaning he was someone who knew how to experimentally manipulate DNA within cells. The shiny new tools of molecular biology promised to blast open the secrets of life and expose the entire genome to explication. We were certain that mutated DNA was the cause of PKD, so it was relatively easy to convince Jim to join the PKD parade, although Sutton's Law may have had a contributing role when he learned that NIH was now pouring money into PKD research, thanks to the activities of the PKRF.

I recruited Ben Cowley, M.D., a newly-issued clinical nephrologist in our training program, to work under the direction of Dr. Calvet to explore the possibility that recently discovered cancer-promoting genes were involved in the relatively aggressive growth of polycystic kidney cells. During the first year of his post-doctoral fellowship, we had the answer — *c-myc* and *c-fos*, *proto-oncogenes* genes associated with cancer, were highly expressed in the kidneys of mice with rapidly progressive PKD. This finding, published in the elite "Proceedings of the National Academy of Science," convinced other scientists throughout the world to enter the PKD field.

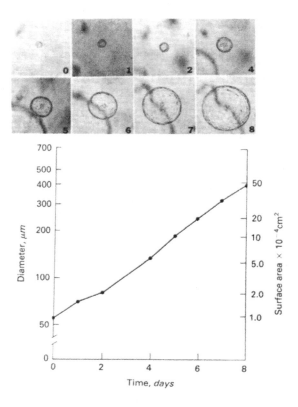

Above. Cyst growing in a Jello-like collagen matrix. MDCK cells were planted in the collagen gel and fed for eight days with nutrients in the medium bathing the gel. One of the cysts that developed is shown in the chart. The diameter of the cyst (scale on the left) increased steadily as a logarithmic function, as did the surface area (on the right). This type of *exponential* growth is similar to that observed in non-malignant tumors.

Our son Aaron had a strong interest in science and had spent several summer vacations working in my lab, assisting others. He was anxious to do his own experiment, so I challenged him to select several micro-cysts in a matrix culture and take careful pictures of them as they enlarged day after day so we could determine how fast their volume increased. This was not an easy thing to do because he had to find a way to identify those cysts he intended to photograph. They all looked like tiny balloons suspended in the air. He might as well have been taking daily photographs of individual penguins in a rookery of hundreds. He figured out a method to track single cysts and took the pictures, which revealed a steady increase in volume from day to day (see Figure).

Aaron made a simple graph starting at day zero in which the logarithm of cyst diameter was plotted against the elapsed time. The dots were connected day-to-day forming a straight line extending over the eight-day experiment. The plot of surface area (right side) and cyst volume (not shown) were straight lines as well, meaning that cyst growth in this model was exponential. The increase in surface area indicated that the cells making up the wall of the cyst were proliferating at a constant rate day to day.

Aaron's finding was explained by a growth process whereby one cell becomes two, four, eight, 16 and so on, indefinitely increasing the surface area of the cyst. The compounding effect of exponential growth explains how cysts can start in renal tubules too small to be seen with the naked eye and over a period of months or years, depending on how fast the cells lining them divide, grow to the size of a grapefruit.

We had little knowledge of what caused these "micro-cysts" to proliferate. I was steered in the right direction to answer this question at a 1988 meeting of the Program Project Grant Steering Committee in Chicago. Greg Everson, M.D. from the University of Colorado was interested in the polycystic liver disease that accompanies ADPKD and was exploring mechanisms by which fluid is secreted into liver cysts. The liver has no glomerular filtration device, so the only way fluid can get into cysts is by secretion. He had found that an intravenous infusion of *secretin*, a hormone that aids in the digestion of protein within the small intestine, increased the secretion of fluid into the liver cysts of a patient with PKD. In the same patient, he injected secretin into the plasma and recorded changes in the volume of a kidney cyst with essentially the same result. I nearly jumped out of my seat when he showed us the data from this study. Secretin is a hormone that stimulates an increase in the level of cyclic AMP, the important "second messenger" within cells that was discussed earlier. Cyclic AMP is a key molecule in the circuit that couple signals from hormones like secretin and vasopressin to the physiological outcome, in this case the secretion of fluid by liver and kidney cysts.

Similar to the clues from a single kidney that led to the discovery of the antibiotic effectiveness of ciprofloxacin in PKD infections, the demonstration in a single kidney cyst that a hormone acting through cyclic AMP stimulated fluid secretion fit with an established paradigm I was caring around in my head. I returned to KUMC after the meeting, anxious to explore more extensively the effects of cyclic AMP-mediated responses to hormones like secretin. Fortunately, Roberto Mangoo-Karim, M.D., a graduate student in Pharmacology, had recently joined the lab to do his Ph.D. thesis work on polycystic kidney disease. I told him I had an inkling that cyclic AMP might be at the heart of cyst growth in PKD and that it would be worth his time to do some exploratory experiments to see if the idea had any merit. We discussed Everson's finding that secretin increased the rate of fluid secretion into a single human kidney cyst; however, I suspected that vasopressin, a.k.a. ADH and AVP, the most prominent cyclic AMP-mediated hormone with actions on the kidney, might be even more important. So we drew up an experiment to determine the effects of vasopressin and secretin on the growth of MDCK micro-cysts in the Jello-like matrix.

The results of the first experiment were clear cut and exciting: Secretin increased the rate of cyst growth by about 30 percent, confirming the effect Everson had observed in the single human cyst. Moreover, vasopressin increased cyst growth by more than 100 percent! In the same experiment, Roberto also demonstrated that vasopressin and the intermediate messenger, cyclic AMP, stimulated cell proliferation as well as fluid secretion, *raising the breathtaking possibility that cell proliferation and fluid secretion, the two most important determinants of cyst growth, may be stimulated by a hormone that is present continuously in blood plasma.*

I had been asked to serve on the Ph.D. thesis committee of William Macias, a graduate student in the Department of Physiology at Indiana University. With his mentor, William Armstrong, Ph.D., Macias discovered that the MDCK cells secreted chloride ions primarily and that sodium ions just went along for the ride. That in itself was an important new fact. But more to my interest, the combined secretory transport of these two ions explained how the liquid part of the secreted fluid was pulled by osmosis through the wall of one of Aaron's *in vitro* microcysts. The Macias discovery implicating chloride, a negatively charged molecule, as the driving force behind the net flow of sodium chloride and water into cysts, was double heresy! Proposing net fluid secretion by renal tubules was one thing, but suggesting that chloride was driving that transport instead of sodium was sure to incite riot among classical renal physiologists as well as my friend Ian Glynn, who had attempted, during my sabbatical in his lab, to convince me that the sodium pump was supreme, admonishing "Thou shalt have no other pumps before me!"

Undaunted, Roberto charged ahead and within a year had completed an impressive study implicating powerful roles for vasopressin and cyclic AMP in the promotion of cyst formation and growth in cysts derived from MDCK cells. The paper was published in the "Proceedings of the National Academy of Sciences" under the sponsorship of my idol and friend, Gerhard Giebisch. There followed studies by Timothy Neufeld, M.D. and Michael Grant, M.D., post-doctoral fellows in the lab, confirming that the MDCK results held true in micro-cysts generated with cells gathered from discarded human kidneys. The increased secretion of salt and water by tubules and cysts in response to vasopressin was now a fact to be reckoned with.

I continued taking regular clinical rotations on the transplant, consultation and dialysis services while administering NIH research grants, Nephrology Division activities, the PKRF and a new position as Councilor of the American Society of Nephrology. On the way home after work one evening, I began seeing two white lines in the middle of the road. No amount of blinking or head turning would resolve the diplopia. I had had no other symptoms of nerve injury or headaches to go along with a brain tumor, and with no pain, infection seemed unlikely. I had been on the kidney transplant service for a month and needed a good night's sleep, so I didn't mention the double vision to Carol, turning in earlier than usual. After an uninterrupted night's sleep, I awoke and still had diplopia, so when I got to work, and with an ophthalmoscope in my hand, I cornered my colleague Dennis Diederich and asked him to check my eyes for papilledema, a sign of brain swelling. He said my eye grounds looked fine, but insisted that I see a neurologist. Dr. Li was just down the hall, so I asked him for a quick consult, and he graciously examined me from stem to stern in his private office. He could find no definite pathology but asked me to get a computed tomogram brain scan just to be on the safe side.

The CT scan revealed that, indeed, I had a brain and that nothing abnormal could be seen. Later in the afternoon, I visited the Chairman of Ophthalmology and sat for an examination that lasted two hours.

"Jared, you have a lazy eye," he reported. "You've been pushing yourself so hard that the abducens muscle in your right eye has pooped out, and you have the equivalent of childhood squint. I'm going to put this temporary plastic lens in your glasses, and it will correct your vision and get rid of the diplopia. And my other prescription is that Carol should take your car keys and not let you out of the house until the muscle flips back and you have normal vision."

I followed his advice and got my vision back after three day's rest. This mini-shaping event signaled me that I had been running faster than my half-body could endure and that it was time to shed some responsibilities. I resigned as Nephrology Director, turning it over to Dr. Diederich. I reduced my clinical service load in order to spend more time in the lab and in clinical studies of PKD. Franz Winklhofer stepped forward to assume responsibility for my patients in the PKD clinic. I continued to serve as founding editor of the "Journal of the American Society of Nephrology," as a council member of the International Society of Nephrology and as a member of the Baker University board of trustees.

I was in Houston giving lectures when word arrived that Allene Bruening had died unexpectedly of a heart attack in her home. Joe was at her side when it happened. He did his best to stay interested and upbeat about the work of the PKRF, but he needed relief when the Executive Director resigned. I stepped in as the interim CEO/President. With the help of Wendy Rueb, the office administrator, and James Martin, our treasurer, we kept things afloat until we could find a new leader. He came in the form of a friend Carol and I had known in our church 20 years earlier. Julian Dyke had just retired from his leadership position with the Boy Scouts of America, headquartered in Dallas, and was persuaded to bring his darling wife, Joanne, with him to Kansas City to help us keep the Foundation moving forward. Julian brought organizational and fundraising skills to bear on our mission and quickly put a fresh plan into action that added money to the treasury sufficient to fund new rounds of individual investigator-initiated grants to researchers across the nation.

I continued to ride an emotional roller coaster. One minute I was on a giddy high having connected some dots that were leading to a potential treatment of PKD only to be jerked downward by the finding that cyclic AMP-dependent fluid secretion into cysts was still not taken seriously by many of my colleagues in renal science. To make matters even worse, one researcher reported that the sodium pump had mistakenly taken aim and was driving sodium into the cysts, not chloride. I decided that we would have to go straight to human cysts to determine the mechanisms of cyst growth if we wanted anyone to believe us. Fortunately, I had just been joined by an urologist on leave from a leading university in Shanghai, China. Ye Min, M.D. was anxious to immerse himself in laboratory research. A gifted surgeon, he developed a method to meticulously dissect individual cysts from the discarded kidneys we procured through a PKRF donation program I had started several years earlier. Soon he had completed an incredible study that we published in the "New England Journal of Medicine" demonstrating that cyclic AMP stimulated fluid secretion into the isolated cysts and that inhibition of the sodium pump from within the cysts was without effect. This study silenced most critics of the chloride section hypothesis as an explanation for the fluid build-up in human renal cysts.

I believe that article was published in a distinguished clinical journal that rarely prints laboratory-based experiments because the associate editor handling our submission was Frank Epstein, M.D., who years earlier had led a team to discover that cyclic AMP stimulated chloride and fluid secretion in the rectal gland of the dogfish shark. Most readers will find connecting shark rectal glands and human renal cysts to be an absurd stretch of credulity; however, it turns out that the cellular mechanisms used by ocean sharks to get rid of extra salt are identical to the ones used to fill human renal cysts. The physician scientist Epstein, excited by this connection when I submitted Ye Min's paper to the "New England Journal of Medicine," saw to it that the manuscript made it safely through the cutthroat review process.

The appearance of this article proving that fluid could be secreted into human renal cysts finally convinced the skeptics that to conserve water, the sacred nephron did more than simply reabsorb it. To advance that heretical view, we needed to discover the cellular and molecular mechanisms that made it possible for salt and water to suddenly switch from being absorbed from the urine to being secreted into it. In this regard, connecting the dots leading from shark rectal glands to human renal cysts illustrates how important it is for research-oriented physicians to work in basic science labs in the course of their training, and conversely, for basic scientists to maintain meaningful contact with physicians who can alert them to potential connections between disease and fundamental mechanisms of no known purpose to man. Discovering that cyclic AMP stimulated chloride secretion in the rectal gland was not only key to eventually determining how renal cysts fill with fluid in PKD, but in understanding why the lungs of children wither and die in children with cystic fibrosis and how cholera toxin provokes massive diarrhea and death in third-world countries.

The mutated gene that causes cystic fibrosis was identified in 1989, and shortly thereafter, the protein encoded by that gene was identified and named CFTR, the abbreviation for Cystic Fibrosis Transmembrane Conductance Regulator. This proved to be a protein that could facilitate the movement of chloride across plasma membranes, and more specifically, to couple the movement of chloride to that of sodium and water, thereby creating a secretory movement of salt and water. In the lungs, the secreted liquid serves as a lubricant making it possible for materials inhaled in the air to be literally carried out of the lungs by cilia on the cells lining the airways. Most individuals notice the product of this normal process upon arising in the mornings when it is often necessary to clear phlegm from the throat. Patients with cystic fibrosis do not have the benefit of this airway clearing system; consequently, bits and pieces of inhaled junk collect deep in the lungs making it possible for bacteria to grow rampantly and destroy lung tissue.

CFTR is also essential for lubricating the cellular surfaces of the small and large intestines; however, when the cholera organism invades the intestines, its toxin abnormally stimulates the production of cyclic AMP causing massive amounts of fluid to be secreted into the gut where it creates disabling dehydration secondary to severe diarrhea. Thus, CFTR, which is a normal membrane protein essential for appropriate pulmonary and intestinal function, can be turned upon the human host by mutations and potent toxins.

I was familiar with the CFTR research because Paul Quinton, Ph.D., who discovered the CFTR mechanism before the actual protein was identified as the defective vagrant in cystic fibrosis, had visited my laboratory in Kansas for several weeks to learn how to perfuse sweat ducts with micropipettes similar to the ones we used to perfuse collecting tubules. CFTR was, therefore, tucked away in my mind, and when we discovered that cysts could secrete chloride and fluid, an unconscious connection somewhere between my eyes was struck to light our path forward.

I had been CEO of the PKRF for five years. Julian Dyke had moved on, and Dan Larson had been recruited to replace him. Under Dan's enthusiastic leadership, private fundraising shot up together with increased funding of grants through the NIH. The PKRF found itself in the delightful position of being petitioned by investigators submitting more exciting studies than it could support. I believed it was time to turn the

Board of Trustees leadership back to a layman with business acumen and asked Tom Flesch, son of Gordon Flesch, one of our early saviors, to lead the crusade against PKD. Tom took charge, and I took leave of PKRF worries, with more time to think about urine rather than raising funds and keeping competing scientists from getting in each others' way.

I was worried about Joe Bruening. He was stuck in an abyss and had lost his sense of humor and interest in almost everything. Carol and I had a secret weapon that we thought might give him reason to rejoin the world. It came in the form of my cousin Peggy, who was more of a sister to me while in our houses in Pratt and Johnson City years earlier. She had been widowed for several years. At a dinner party one evening, I was teasing her about why such a pretty lady remained unattached, and she retorted, "Well, I'm waiting for you to find me a rich one!"

So we invited Joe to have dinner with us in our home, and we asked Peggy to "round out the table." They hit it off, and as Carol was clearing the table before serving dessert, Joe announced that he and Peggy were going to the Plaza to have dessert and listen to jazz. They started seeing each other regularly, and after about a year of courtship, Joe proposed and Peggy accepted. Just like that, Joe and I became cousins.

Larry Sullivan, Ph.D., who taught the Renal Physiology course for medical students at KUMC, and I entered a collaboration in the early 1990s to explore the mechanisms of sodium, chloride and water transport across kidney tubules. Larry had hired Darren P. Wallace, a bright young technician to work on the projects, and it soon became clear that the "technician" was not just twisting dials but making impressive methodological innovations. Wallace was eventually recruited into the graduate program where his prodigious talent for research could be used to satisfy requirements for a Ph.D. in Physiology. Together, we set on a path to define the molecular basis of chloride and fluid secretion in the epithelia derived from human renal cysts. We were joined along the way by Tamio Yamaguchi, Ph.D. and Clarissa Davidow, Ph.D. at KUMC and Michael Caplan, Ph.D. at Yale in a wonderfully collaborative series of experiments proving that CFTR, the chloride channel that fails to work in cystic fibrosis, was over-working in the cells lining renal cysts. Chloride moved in abnormal amounts through the channels created by excess CFTR in the cells lining the cysts causing sodium and water to rush across as well. And as our hypothesis forecast, the secretion of chloride-rich fluid into the cysts was stimulated by cyclic AMP to a striking degree.

Tamio Yamaguchi, Ph.D., a skilled experimentalist, was given the task of determining if cyclic AMP and its agonist, vasopressin, also promoted the growth of cells removed from the cysts of patients with ADPKD. In an elegant series of experiments, he showed that cyclic AMP and vasopressin stimulated the proliferation of cells removed from human polycystic kidneys, confirming another hypothesis borrowed from our MDCK work. Researchers at Johns Hopkins University, who also examined human kidney tissues, corroborated Yamaguchi's findings. This discovery strengthened the claim that cyclic AMP played a central role in the enlargement of cysts and kidneys in ADPKD. Now, we had in hand a hormone messenger capable of regulating both major elements responsible for cyst growth: the number of mural cells determined by proliferation and the secretion of fluid into the potential space formed by the expanding wall. Moreover, now we had clearly defined targets for an attack to prevent, slow or eradicate renal cysts in ADPKD.

CHAPTER 29

It's water, stupid!

Animals that live on dry land must conserve water to survive; however, the kidneys have to excrete enough water to get rid of the unwanted metabolic debris, environmental toxins and excess dietary minerals that are disposed of in the urine. Normal persons eating a well-balanced diet need to excrete about 500 milliliters (1 pint, 16 ounces) of urine each day. This volume is the least amount that would be needed to eliminate waste molecules that have been maximally concentrated in the urine. Normal human kidneys can concentrate the urinary solutes about three to four times greater than the plasma. The elegant biological mechanisms that operate to maximally concentrate the urine come at a high cost to patients with ADPKD because high plasma concentrations of the anti-diuretic hormone (vasopressin) are required.

Since normal humans drink fluids irregularly, usually to slake thirst, the kidneys spend most of the day and night conserving water.

Consequently, vasopressin generates cyclic AMP in the cells of normal persons and those with PKD nearly 24 hours a day! As it is supposed to do in normal people! But as we have learned, this process is bad for polycystic kidneys because it makes the cysts and the kidneys enlarge above normal size. Knowing this bad stuff about vasopressin in PKD, Vincent Gattone, Ph.D. at KUMC obtained a new chemical, OPC-31260, from the Otsuka Pharmaceutical Corporation of Japan (OPCJ) that blocked the action of the hormone in the kidney. OPC-31260, a chemical under investigation by the company, was known to block the capacity of vasopressin to bind to a highly selective spot (AVP-V2 receptor) on the surface of renal tubules called collecting ducts. Collecting ducts, the last kidney tubule segments urine passes through on the way to the urinary bladder, regulate water excretion. Imagine that a molecule of water bumps into the wall of a collecting duct cell containing a door through which it could pass to get to the other side of the cell, but the door is closed. The door has a keyhole, a receptor that can open the door if a proper key fits in the keyhole. Vasopressin turns out to be the key that fits into the keyhole and the door swings open, letting the water molecule pass to the other side. In this way, vasopressin opens the door and water flows from the urine back into the blood, thus saving the water and concentrating the solutes left behind in the urine.

OPC-31260 is actually an impotent vasopressin molecule that acts like a receptor blocker; it bears enough resemblance to the hormone to get into the keyhole receptor easily. However, it cannot activate the other mechanisms needed to open the door. As long as OPC-31260 sits in the keyhole, vasopressin is blocked from getting in; consequently, the door remains closed and water molecules can't get through and are lost into the urine rather than being absorbed back into the blood. When OPC-31260 was given to experimental animals, it caused them to urinate profusely and become thirsty, requiring them to drink more water.

Gattone reasoned that giving animals OPC-31260 would reduce the effect of vasopressin on the cysts. He knew that this drug would also increase thirst and water intake, but he believed that increased urination would be a price worth paying if the drug reduced the size of the kidneys and slowed the rate of kidney function decline. He performed a key experiment in mice with a rapidly progressive type of PKD that usually causes death within three weeks after birth. The results were strikingly positive: Animals that received OPC-31260 had smaller kidneys, better renal function and survived longer than animals that were not treated. Gattone had hit a colossal home run, prompting him to apply for and receive a "use" patent for drugs like OPC-31260 that might be developed to treat PKD.

There was a formidable barrier to clinical trials that had to be breeched before any drug could be tried in patients with ADPKD. The cysts begin to form in the affected fetus and throughout the patient's lifetime. Once formed, they enlarge progressively, driven day and night by vasopressin. The disease announces its presence as early as childhood in a few patients through the development of bloody urine, as my friend Ronnie had experienced, or through the development of high blood pressure or by moderate to severe pain in the flanks. Some women don't learn they have ADPKD until they have their first fetal ultrasound and are told that the baby is fine, but the expectant mother has cysts in the kidneys. Eventually the cysts become numerous and damage kidney function; at this point, usually in the fifth or sixth decade of life, routine lab tests reveal an increase in the serum creatinine concentration, alerting physicians that renal function is in decline.

ADPKD begins to cause the loss of functioning nephrons early in the course of the disease; however, the usual indicators (biomarkers) of kidney function, serum creatinine and urea, do not begin to rise until about one-half of the kidney mass has been turned into scar tissue. The kidneys have a remarkable capacity to compensate for the loss of functioning tissue, a fact we see play out when one person donates a kidney to another. When we take a normal organ and give it to someone whose kidneys have been destroyed by disease, the donor is left with only 50 percent of the usual plasma filtering capacity. In other words, shortly after the operation, both the donor and the recipient have "renal insufficiency." However, when we check kidney function a year later, we find that that the serum creatinine and urea levels are only slightly higher than the values the donor had before the surgery. The residual kidney in the donor has not grown new nephrons; rather, each remaining nephron has been stimulated to work twice as hard as before to keep chemicals in the blood plasma at levels we would consider normal. This complex and scientifically mysterious post-nephrectomy process affecting the nephrons is called renal compensation.

This same compensation process is at work in patients with polycystic kidneys where the functioning nephrons are deleted one at a time, rather than all at once as in renal donation. When one nephron out of the one million in each kidney is destroyed by the disease, another normal nephron pitches in and works twice as hard to keep overall renal function within normal limits. In other words, the compensation process that operates "wholesale" in kidney donation works the same magic — "retail" — approximately one nephron at a time in slowly progressive cystic disease. This process repeats itself each time a normal nephron is lost to the disease until a point is finally reached where all of the nephrons are working at least double time and unable to work any harder. As the cystic disease continues to march along, the double-duty nephrons are also destroyed, making it impossible for the kidney to keep up with the body's production of creatinine; consequently, the plasma creatinine levels rise signaling that renal function is declining toward the end stage.

Unfortunately, the rise in the serum creatinine concentration is a relatively late sign of disease progression, and by the time it climbs high enough to be clearly abnormal, more than 50 percent of kidney function has been lost. This would not be the best time to start treating patients with a drug targeting cyclic AMP dependent cell proliferation and fluid secretion, as the medication will not touch the secondary fibrosis and inflammation components that comprise the end-stage-disease program. We needed a marker of disease progression that could be accurately measured in the early stages of the disease, before major damage had been done.

It occurred to me that since cysts were in fact renal tumors, we might measure kidney and cyst volume repeatedly to determine their rates of growth, just like cancer doctors do when following the growth of a lung or brain tumor. I enlisted the help of a renal fellow, Cori Sise, M.D., and a visiting trainee from Japan, Tomo Kusaka, to measure changes in total kidney volume by computed tomography in patients we had followed in the PKD clinic for several years. Unknown to me, Vicente Torres, M.D. and Bernard King, M.D. at the Mayo Clinic had the same idea and had prospectively obtained kidney volume data on several ADPKD patients. The results of these pilot studies showed that kidney volume increased from year to year in what appeared to be a predictable pattern; moreover, those patients with the largest kidneys were the most likely to develop kidney malfunction.

I contacted Josephine Briggs, M.D., Director of the Kidney, Urology and Hematology Program at the NIH, and implored her to support an imaging study to determine in 200 to 300 patients with ADPKD if the rate of kidney growth was a satisfactory indicator of disease progression. She listened politely, but I could tell she was not enthused. Here I was trying to get her to invest millions of dollars in a project most renal scientists would label "blue collar" or, more devastatingly, "uninteresting." NIH is committed to keeping the United States on the cutting edge of medical science, which for most scientists means molecular research involving DNA, RNA, cloned genes and stem cells. Those topics are gleaming sports cars when viewed against a Model T concept like determining how fast kidneys grow. We marshaled the persuasive forces of the newly renamed Polycystic Kidney Disease Foundation to lean on the NIH with the help of several friendly senators and congresspersons who made phone calls to "encourage" Dr. Briggs and her boss to make the PKD study happen. I don't think Josie ever forgave me for the arm-twisting, but the NIH finally came around and assigned James Scherbenske, Ph.D. (the KUH administrator who helped start it all years earlier) to write the request for proposals announcement that would go to research centers across the nation.

The day before the request for proposals to measure kidney volume went out from the NIH, Josie called me and said firmly, "Jared, I'm going to take a lot of heat from the molecular scientists we can't fund because we are putting so much money into measuring kidney volume. Can you assure me that this is going to work?"

I remember my reply: "Josie, I'm looking as we speak at data from our retrospective study, and I can assure you that based on the cases we have examined together with those Torres has studied at Mayo, this is going to work."

She seemed satisfied with my assurance and then said goodbye, probably wondering if she was about to sign her ticket to administrative oblivion.

Several institutions responded to the NIH request for proposals and spanning a period of several months, the Mayo Clinic, Emory University, The University of Alabama and The University of Kansas were selected to do the study using frontline kidney imaging technology to document changes in kidney volume in approximately 250 patients with autosomal dominant PKD (ADPKD). Washington University in St. Louis was selected to be the data collection and statistical analysis center and K. Ty Bae, M.D., Ph.D., an innovative radiologist at the same institution, was selected to develop the magnetic resonance imaging (MRI) protocol for determining kidney volume. The nickname given to this project, CRISP, was derived from the longer title: Consortium for Radiologic Imaging Studies of Polycystic Kidney Disease.

The type of funding mechanism used in such multicenter projects is called an U01, which is NIH code for administrative chaos. In our first meeting on the NIH campus in Washington, representatives from the five institutions were brought together, without a leader being named, and asked to produce a detailed protocol before we had decided just exactly what we would be doing and how we were going to do it. Every institutional representative in this consortium was accustomed to being in charge, so the first meeting consisted largely of arguing points of view, jousting and throwing up ideas, and catching the good ones before they fell to the floor. We managed to agree to meet again by electronic conferencing and face-to-face meetings to hash out the formal protocols for the study and for writing the detailed informed consent documents we would have to submit to our institutional human subjects review boards for approval. It took about a year to finish the initial task; from there, we were off and running.

We enrolled 241 volunteers who agreed to have magnetic resonance imaging (MRI) studies done annually over a period of four years as well as measurements of kidney function that required multiple blood samples and urine collections. At KU, I hired two nurses to work on the project, Jody Mahan and Beth Stafford, who had been standout caregivers in our renal dialysis unit. They were very comfortable communicating with patients and soon we had more than 80 volunteers signed up. I recruited three co-investigators at Kansas: Louis Wetzel, M.D., Professor of Radiology, who would manage the MR studies that had to be done to exacting standards; Franz Winklhofer, M.D., Assistant Professor of Medicine/Nephrology, who supervised a large polycystic kidney clinic; and physicist Larry Cook, Ph.D., who helped process the MR images and develop mathematical models of kidney enlargement. In order to standardize methods, four of the volunteers, one from each participating center, stepped forward to have the MRI and kidney function measurements done at each of the four sites. This willingness to move things forward illustrates the importance and the urgency that patients with this disease put on gaining new knowledge, especially when it has the potential to improve treatment to avoid kidney failure.

At the Kansas PKD Center in the 1990s, we had our eyes on potential treatments for ADPKD. We had discovered that the renal inflammation associated with the disease could be suppressed and the rate of kidney enlargement decreased by drugs currently available to patients: methylprednisolone, a potent anti-inflammatory compound, and lovastatin, a cholesterol-lowering agent. In other words, proof of principle had been established for these drugs, inviting the development of better agents more specifically targeting ADPKD. I had contacted several pharmaceutical companies, hoping to develop their interest in adding ADPKD to the list of disorders they sought to treat. Only one company, Merck, invited me to their research center to discuss an anti-cancer compound they had under study that was a more potent version of lovastatin.

In my research presentation to the Merck scientists and administrators, I emphasized that lovastatin, a farnesyltransferase inhibitor like the more potent agent they were developing, had significantly slowed the progression of ADPKD in rats with the disease. We were interested in administering their more potent compound to polycystic animals to see if it might be even more effective than lovastatin. The response from the laboratory group was cordial but tepid. As I was ushered out the door of the Merck vice-president's office, my last meeting of the day, he told me that he was not interested in any further discussions with me or anyone working on ADPKD. Ouch! That stung. Damn these "Dangerfield Disorders!"

I limped home wondering if we would ever find a willing partner in this industry. A few weeks later, I received an email from David Woo, Ph.D., a PKD scientist in San Francisco, alerting me that in a new patent application for a farnesyltranferase inhibitor, Merck had included ADPKD in its list of potential diseases that might benefit from the drug. Well, I hadn't flunked out completely. Incidentally, the Merck drug never made it to the clinic; on the other hand, University of Colorado researchers reported recently that a cholesterol-lowering drug resembling lovastatin reduced the growth and the rate of functional decline in children with ADPKD.

Fortunately, I got a nice pat-on-the-back from an unexpected source. To honor his mother, a victim of ADPKD, in 2003 Thomas Kaplan established the Lillian Jean Kaplan Prize for Advancement in the Understanding of Polycystic Kidney Disease. He enlisted the International Society of Nephrology and the Polycystic Kidney Disease Foundation to recruit a select advisory panel to choose among scientists who had made the strongest contribution to the body of knowledge in the PKD field. Peter Harris, Mayo Clinic, and I were chosen to receive the inaugural awards at a symposium on PKD held during the 2003 meeting of the International Society of Nephrology in Berlin, Germany. Since then, 10 more Kaplan laureates have been named and feted, repeatedly exposing the broad scientific community to the robust progress being made in understanding polycystic kidney disorders.

Vince Gattone's pivotal experiment in 1999 and later move to Indiana University preceded his collaboration with Vicente Torres to test OPC-31260 (mozavaptan) in other animal models of PKD. The drug proved to be effective in two disparate models of PKD, leading to an abstract they presented at the 2003 annual conference of the American Society of Nephrology. They had contacted the Otsuka Pharmaceutical Corporation of Japan (OPCJ) and were to meet with company representatives at some time after the meeting. Fortuitously, Frank Czerwiec, M.D., Ph.D., Senior Director for Otsuka's Global Clinical Development group, attended the OPC-31260 presentation, unaware of their work or that they had contacted OPCJ. At that meeting, Czerweic met and conversed with Gattone, Torres and Dan Larson, the President of the Polycystic Kidney Disease Foundation, beginning a dialog about how a clinical trial might proceed. Czerweic's bosses at Otsuka, Rockville, Maryland, Cesare Orlandi, M.D. and Junichi Kamabyashi, M.D., Ph.D. were onboard right away.

Those of us who had labored in this field for decades agreed that the time was right to strongly encourage the OPCJ to conduct a formal trial in patients with ADPKD. OPJC representatives visited Indiana University, Mayo Clinic and Kansas University where they were warmly received. It was Toyoki Mori, Ph.D. from Japan's Otsuka Corporation Tokushima Research Institute who visited my laboratory for the purpose of discussing the potential treatment of ADPKD patients. He informed me that any trial would be done with OPC-41061 (tolvaptan), a more specific vasopressin inhibitor than OPC-31260. The company had initiated several international, Phase III clinical trials to determine if tolvaptan would help the kidneys get rid of extra water in patients with low levels of salt in their blood (hyponatremia) and in a huge trial for patients with excess water in their lungs and other tissues due to congestive heart failure (CHF). The toxicity tests, Phase I and Phase II trials had been done, so repurposing tolvaptan would mean the drug had a head start in a study involving ADPKD patients.

I arranged for Dr. Mori to visit the home office of the PKDF in Kansas City, Missouri, where the president and members of his staff welcomed him. In this meeting, Dr. Mori gained a perspective on how many potential volunteers might be available in the United States for a large clinical trial.

Studies such as these are frightfully expensive and must be done before agencies, such as the federal Food and Drug Administration (FDA), will approve a new drug for sale to patients. Several years and many meetings with the FDA are often required just to approve the protocol that will be used to test the candidate drug's efficacy. The company sponsoring the drug must do an elaborate series of tests to show that it will not cause cancer, organ injury or build up in the body to harmful levels. In the pre-clinical phase, drugs are screened in animals looking for candidates that might work in specific diseases. Once a compound is identified, potential toxic effects are tested in animals and living tissues, such as cell culture, and dosage levels are determined.

Once the drug passes these checks, it enters Phase I testing in a few human volunteers to see how well it is tolerated and how it is processed in the human body. If it is tolerated well, the drug passes into Phase II and a larger number of volunteers are tested to see if it performs as proposed. If drug efficacy is demonstrated and toxic effects are minimal, it passes into the gold standard trial called Phase III, which usually uses the "double-blind, placebo-controlled" design in several hundred to several thousand patients over approximately three years to verify any positive effect it may have on the course of the disease. It is not uncommon to spend a billion dollars bringing a new drug through this process — and sadly, in this ordeal, more new drugs are proven to not be beneficial in humans than advance to clinical use.

Vicente Torres and I were invited to visit the Otsuka Tokushima Research Institute in Japan on separate occasions where we met corporate officers and working scientists, all of who had penetrating questions about a possible clinical trial. On reflection, I can't fault their due diligence as they were considering investing hundreds of millions of dollars in an idea some wild guys in America had come up with. Had it been my company, I would probably have administered lie detection tests as well.

The discovery of new drugs and their eventual application to a disease does not usually proceed this way, but remember, this is PKD — a "Dangerfield Disorder" — and conventional rituals do not apply. Unlike cardiologists and oncologists, who are pursued by the NIH and pharmaceutical companies with grants and drugs in hand, PKD researchers usually have to beg for grants from the NIH and plead for support from pharmaceutical companies. Although we appeared to have a friend in OPCJ, we took nothing for granted, working persistently to reach the goal of a full-scale pivotal trial. In retrospect, we could have been more at ease. I have since learned from two sources that Mr. Akihiko Otsuka, the Chairman of OPJC, a privately held company at the time, had stated to effect: "We must test our drugs for the disease, not because it would be profitable, but because these patients have no available options."

In the interest of full disclosure, I became a consultant to the Otsuka Corporation specifically to help with the design and analysis of treatment protocols. I accepted reimbursement for travel and a stipend based on the amount of time I spent working on the project. Years earlier, Vincent Gattone and the University of Kansas had received a patent covering the use of vasopressin-receptor inhibitors in the treatment of PKD; no other individual at the University of Kansas was party to the patent.

Based on our preliminary studies, slowing total kidney volume was selected as the primary outcome of a clinical trial. The CRISP study was just finishing the first phase of funding and sufficient data was collected from the 241 enrollees in the study to write the initial report describing the change in total kidney volume over time and the relation of kidney volume to declining renal function. I was chosen to organize the data and write a draft manuscript that would eventually be submitted to the

"New England Journal of Medicine." As the data had been unfolding, I had plotted a graph of the total kidney volumes that connected the dots of individual patients, beginning at baseline, with those at one, two and three years. The baseline kidney volumes varied widely from subject to subject, so the lines that followed the baseline were scattered about as well. Yet, nearly all of the kidney volumes, and the lines connecting them, increased with time. The mass of data obscured the message to anyone who stared intently at it for hours on end. When I showed this very busy graph to some of my colleagues at KUMC, they suggested that I start looking for another job. On a lark, one day I showed the graph to my grandson, Connor, when he was visiting. He was a junior in high school and had set his sights on a career in medicine.

"What's this data set look like to you, Connor?" I asked, knowing that he had recently taken calculus in an advanced placement class.

He looked at it and asked a couple of questions, then said, "It looks like an exponential, Grandpa."

When I turned my eyes to the screen, I was immediately struck by the pattern of lines now that the word "exponential" had been said aloud.

"Damned if it's not!" I replied.

What Connor's unbiased eyes had seen was the upsweep of the individual curves, an augenblick recognition moment that happens frequently in the practice of medicine; a consultant will walk into a patient's room and render an instant diagnosis that had escaped equally observant physicians who had been there day after day. Recognizing the exponential shape of the kidney growth curves provided strong confirmatory evidence that the organs in human subjects were growing just like those individual cysts Connor's father, Aaron, had grown and measured in an artificial environment more than two decades before. The MRI study also revealed that both kidneys in a patient were expanding at about the same rate; thus, it was logical to suppose that the individual cysts within the kidneys must also be programmed to expand in concert in order to generate a predictable growth curve maintained across several years. It followed that the processes controlling the rate of cyst

— as well as kidney — growth must be inherent and constant features residing within each cyst.

One of the best examples of the power of exponential growth is the compound interest investors seek on certificates of deposits (CD) and savings accounts. With compounding, the total value increases more than when invested at simple interest because each day we earn interest on the accumulated interest as well as the amount invested. The value of a CD earning 8 percent compound interest will double the amount initially invested within nine years; by contrast, simple interest of 8 percent for nine years would be worth only 1.72 times the original investment. Similarly, kidneys growing exponentially at the rate of 8 percent per year will be twice as large after nine years and only 1.72 times as large after nine years in the absence of compounding.

One of the puzzling mysteries about ADPKD was the recognition that patients with the most common genetic type, PKD1, had larger kidneys and developed kidney failure at a younger age than those with PKD2. A secondary analysis of the MRI study provided an explanation for this difference: Those patients with PKD2 have fewer renal cysts than those with PKD1. This finding suggested that overall kidney size depends on the number of cysts as well as the collective rate at which the cysts grow. The study also revealed the surprising finding that the PKD1 and PKD2 kidneys grew at about the same annual rate even though the PKD1 kidneys were about twice as large as those in PKD2. The simple answer to this teaser is that more cysts growing at the same rate yield larger kidneys growing at the same rate. The MRI study increased our fundamental understanding of cyst formation and cyst growth and set the stage for the use of total kidney volume, kidney growth rate, and total cyst number to determine in clinical trials if that inherent rate of cyst growth that typifies each ADPKD patient's kidneys can be modified by diet or pharmacologic treatment.

❖

CHAPTER 30

Another bump in the road

Josie Briggs, our reluctant champion at the NIH, slept a little easier as she watched the data from the MRI study falling into place and meeting more than our original expectations. The study proved to be a treasure-trove of new facts and insights that had escaped consideration in our ignorance. Out of this initially disorganized, polarized, passionate brew of PKD clinicians and radiologists bubbled up an elegantly simple technology with the potential to divine the future course of ADPKD in individual patients beginning as early as childhood. It was a doubly-thrilling adventure for me to watch a "blue collar" idea blossom into findings worthy of report in, arguably, the top clinical medical journal in the world, "The New England Journal of Medicine."

The Steering Committee for the study included the active participants: Vicente Torres, M.D., Arlene Chapman, M.D., Lisa Guay-Woodford, M.D., Kyongtae Bae, M.D., Ph.D., Bernard King, M.D., Louis Wetzel, M.D., Peter Harris, Ph.D., John Miller, A.B., William Bennett, M.D. and myself. I was assigned the task of writing the draft of the manuscript based on the quantitative information that poured in from a complex statistical analysis. We haggled through several revisions until everyone was finally satisfied with the version we sent to the journal for consideration. The turnaround was quick, and editor Julie Ingelfinger's comments were encouraging that it might be published. But, true to the practice of this journal, three anonymous reviewers had posted a long list of questions and challenges that the other co-authors and I had to deal with. I went to work on the revision at once.

It was the dead of winter, and I was ready to take a short break from revising the MRI paper. The day February 7, 2006, had been brightened by a visit from Shizuko Nagao, Ph.D. from Toyoake, Japan, who had spent several months in the KU laboratory a few years earlier. She had returned to Japan to continue her work on PKD in experimental animals, one of which had been developed by my friend Hisehida Takahashi Ph.D., who had visited Kansas City several years earlier to establish a fruitful collaboration. Tamio Yamaguchi, Ph.D., a former member of the Takahashi lab, had done his thesis work under my direction and was now a faculty member in the Kidney Institute at KUMC. He and Darren Wallace joined Shizuko and me for lunch at a quiet restaurant two blocks east of the campus on 39th Street. After our grand reunion, I broke away to visit the library directly across the street from the lab, heading to the stacks on the second floor to look up a reference.

The last thing I remember was sliding and bumping headlong down the stairs unable to move my arms or legs. My last thoughts were, "Oh shit! This isn't good," followed by a sanguine feeling that dying wasn't so bad after all. Much later, I opened my eyes and through a haze saw my son Aaron and daughter, Janeane, looking down at me. I could not speak because a ventilator tube had been crammed up my nose and into my trachea. In the other nostril, a plastic tube had been threaded into my stomach to infuse water, medications and liquid food.

I could hear Aaron speaking to me, something about breaking my neck yesterday. There was a very sore spot on the left side of my head. I knew something was amiss, as I could not move either arm and only wiggle the fingers of my right hand; both arms and hands were numb. I could move both legs a little, but they, too, were numb. My mind was clearing rapidly, and I was aware that higher ordered brain functions were intact, if a bit fuzzy. "Strange broken neck," I thought to myself. "Legs working better than arms."

Aaron was trying to get my attention. When I finally finished my own physical inventory, I looked squarely at him. He asked me to blink my right eye when he reached the correct letter as he went through the alphabet repeatedly, a technique most physicians learn in order to communicate with quadriplegic patients on ventilators. In short order, I spelled out M-I-N-D G-O-O-D, and I could hear a cheer go up from others in the room including Carol who pushed her way past the others to plant a kiss on my forehead. Taylor was the next to welcome me back to planet Earth from wherever I had been for the last day and a half.

Later, I reconstructed the event from interviews with those who were on the scene. Evidently, when I finished whatever I had come to the library to do, I walked toward the stairway leading down to the main floor. I failed to see an unmarked step-down about 3 inches in height that created a false floor under which computer cables were run to several stations. I had tripped, lunging forward toward the stairs. Ordinary persons would reach out and avoid driving their heads, powered by 200 pounds of carcass, into the brick wall onto which the handrails were attached. Since polio residual kept me from raising my arms, I hit the wall with the left side of my skull full force, abruptly forcing my head sideways and crushing the 4th and 5th vertebrae in my neck. I was saved from a spinal transection by virtue of a previous shaping experience requiring that the bones in my neck be fused. Rather than being completely quadriplegic, the fusion held part of the neck together enough to keep the spinal cord from tearing; instead, it was bounced from one side of the spinal column to the next, creating what is called a central cord lesion, which the neurological hospitalist diagnosed immediately when he discovered that my legs were better off than my arms. It turns out the arm nerves travel near the center of the spinal cord and the legs closer to the edge. The central part of the cord took the heaviest shock when I bounced against the wall.

It was bad enough, in any event, to kill me, as I had stopped breathing and was deep blue turning to black when two surgery residents came to help. Weesam Al-Khatib, M.D., resident in plastic surgery, and Amir Nassir, M.D., resident in general surgery, had been reading in the library and heard me fall on the steps. They raced to the stairs and saw immediately that I had a serious neck injury as my head was displaced to the side at a severe angle. Two students arrived to help: Lorelei Witt, R.N., nurse practitioner, and Katherine Humphrey, nursing student and former respiratory therapist. Together, this quartet logrolled me onto my back and positioned me on the first landing where Waseem did mouth-to-mouth respiration and chest compression. Amir summoned the ambulance. Elizabeth Banks, the librarian at the front desk and former emergency medical therapist, happened to have an oral airway in her purse that Katherine applied, improving pulmonary ventilation and quickly "pinking" me up. They were able to keep me stable until the ambulance arrived.

Growing up in a racially and ethnically "pure" village in western Kansas did not prepare me for the smorgasbord of people I would encounter later in life, and I had to fight continuously to suppress my congenital racism. Thankfully, experiences at Baker University, the National Institutes of Health, The University of Kansas Medical Center and The Methodist Church had armed me with the will and the tools to embrace those different from myself in all walks of life. Here on the steps of Dykes Library, my conversion from bigotry was rewarded when two Muslim men of Middle East descent whose families emigrated from Iraq and Pakistan gave me back my life.

My family was called to the hospital and gathered in the emergency room awaiting news about what was going on. Carol sat with me and insists that I was conscious and communicating with eye movements, but that is lost to me. I ended up with four broken ribs, a head contusion, a false aneurysm in my left femoral artery that was fixed several days later, two crushed cervical vertebrae and extremities that weren't worth much to begin with because of post-polio syndrome and now were simply props.

Chris Glattes, M.D. was called in to do the surgery. One thing about staying in your home institution for an entire career is that you know the scene pretty well. I had classmates and collaborators in key departments throughout the medical center, including a spine surgeon and classmate who wrote the book on fixing scoliosis in children. Marc Asher, M.D. appeared as though mystically summoned to reassure Carol and my children that he would trust Dr. Glattes to operate on any member of his family. The surgery to stabilize what was left of my spine took nine hours and required bone grafts, rods, bolts and wire. I was placed in a "halo," a device that rests on the shoulders, chest and back and impales the head through four stainless steel spikes that are literally screwed through the scalp to hold the head perfectly still. I got to wear this thing for 90 days.

The tubes came out of my lungs and stomach in a couple of days, and the remaining postoperative period was uneventful save for the horrible constipation that is caused when oxycontin, the pain killer, paralyzes the bowels. A nurse named Cynthia introduced me to "Cynthia's cocktail" — an ounce of milk of magnesia, two ounces of prune juice and three tablespoons of melted butter drunk at one setting — which she guaranteed would clean me out by 4 pm if I drank it at 8 am. I asked her to "bring it on." I took the stuff at 8 am, and I could have set my watch by the explosion at 4 pm. Cynthia had won my deep affection.

I told my doctor son, Aaron, about the wonder brew, but he was not amused. "Why are you taking oxycontin?" he snarled.

"Because I hurt, I guess." I have to admit that I felt pretty good taking the stuff. Visitors would marvel at how spirited I seemed. Darren Wallace visited, and I told him about four new experiments I thought he should do. On thinking back, I believe he faked a cell phone call so he could get out of the room. Upon Aaron's insistence, I had them discontinue the oxycontin.

Soon the reality of enforced rehabilitation fell upon me. I had sessions with occupational and physical therapists twice a day. I was beginning to get more movement in my right hand, and I could move the thumb of the left hand a little. Otherwise my arms were numb, dead weight. At night, I had severe, burning pains in my left arm and hand requiring Tylenol or something stronger from time to time. I learned that I had a type of pain called complex regional pain syndrome, abbreviated CRPS. Neurologists had described it as pain appearing after severe spinal cord or peripheral nerve injuries, but no one had any idea of the specific cause or how to treat it. After suffering with it for several weeks, I renamed it complex regional aggravating pain syndrome, abbreviated CRAPS and wrote a letter about it, which the "New England Journal" did not see fit to print.

Speaking of the "New England Journal," Vicente Torres pitched in and finished answering the reviewer's critiques and rendered the CRISP paper acceptable for publication. Barry Brenner, M.D., whom I had known since our fellowship days at the NIH, called me in the hospital one day to admonish me for not getting my textbook chapter on PKD in on time. I had written that chapter for his classic text for nearly 30 years.

"But Barry, how can I write the chapter? I can't even wipe my ass," I cried.

"Get Carol to type it as you dictate. What else do you have to do for the next 90 days?" came the reply.

After the patter died down, I told Barry that I would con Vicente Torres into updating the PKD chapter with the understanding that Torres would become the lead author. Dropping his curmudgeon act for a moment, he agreed that my suggestion was an easy solution.

Over the next three weeks, I got up on my feet and relearned how to walk. I had numb feet that made things interesting, especially in the dark. There were encouraging signs of recovery in my right hand, but the left was balking as well as hurting. The occupational therapists have clever ways of getting your hands to work for you, but invariably, there is some discomfort or outright pain involved. The physical therapists are not as cunning — they just grab and bend and twist until they see tears or are stopped by an armed threat. In a hospital rehabilitation unit, you can expect to find angels (aides), saints (nurses) and beasts with smiling faces.

After four weeks in the hospital, I was discharged home to continue occupational and physical therapy. We also engaged a home health agency to help me get started in the morning and made ready for sleep at night. I spent most of the time in a reclining chair in the great room where I could watch television. The pain in my left arm and hand was so intense at times that Carol would have to do gentle massage late into the evening before I got relief. I was reluctant to use narcotics and tried to use the next best things as much as I could. My rehab doctor at KU finally set me up for more intensive daily occupational therapy at the Rehabilitation Institute in downtown Kansas City. To relieve Carol, several of my male friends, including Les Holdeman, Paul Schloerb and Larry Sullivan, took turns driving the 10 miles to the rehab center. Gradually, the left hand and arm came around, and I could use the computer.

I wrote my first note to friends using the index fingers of both hands on one of the days when I was feeling a little sorry for myself.

> Dear friends,
>
> We've been home for three weeks.
>
> Steady stream of cars coming to house. Therapists and visitors.
>
> Visitors are very welcome. Therapists bring pain.
>
> Rumors in neighborhood that we sell Amway products or deal drugs.
>
> To confuse matters, the physical therapist puts a large belt on me around waist, which is attached to a leash. She then walks me for 10 minutes up and down the driveway.
>
> In my halo, I look like a captured Martian or some kind of a unique, muzzled animal.
>
> Still waiting for arms to come around.
>
> Summing things up at this point of rehab, I would say that at the worst, I will make a good pet for Carol.
>
> Better than a pet rock because I can walk.
>
> As good as or better than a cat because I can talk.
>
> And better than a dog because I can poop on command.

With any luck, I may yet advance to full human companion status.

Cheers.

Jared

After 90 days, the halo came off, and I felt like I had been freed from the ball and chain. My walking resembled that of a tipsy sailor on leave, and still does, but my steps became more certain each day. The high point came when I took a rigorous driving test at the Rehabilitation Institute and passed. Now I could drive myself to rehab for treatments and give some thought to returning to work. Since I was covered under the workers compensation law, it was necessary to get a formal rating on the degree of disability. I checked out at 33 percent whole, which is better than it might have been had the old spinal fusion not given me a modicum of protection.

Things were looking up, and my mind lifted thoughts about urine back to the highest priority.

CHAPTER 31

This drug will drive you to drink

Rescue from my assignation with eternity kept me in the project to test the potential of tolvaptan to slow the course of ADPKD in patients. In 2004, investigator sites had been spotted in the United States and Japan, and volunteers were recruited for several Phase II trials to establish potential efficacy and to reveal any side effects that tolvaptan might cause with prolonged use. With the recent publication in the "New England Journal" confirming that kidney volume was a dependable marker of disease progression, consultants to and research staff in the Otsuka Pharmaceutical Global Clinical Development group, Rockville, Marlyand, agreed that Total Kidney Volume (TKV) was an ideal marker of disease progression. Enlarged kidneys are the hallmark of ADPKD; patients would undoubtedly welcome a drug that curbed the bloated abdomen; an added bonus would be slowing the loss of function.

ADPKD causes undetected kidney injury as early as infancy in some. Because the normal nephrons are called on to work harder as cystic nephrons are shut down, doctors usually do not see evidence of kidney malfunction until nearly one-half of the blood filters have been destroyed. That point is usually not reached until the fifth or sixth decades of life when serum creatinine levels rise above normal. Because the serum creatinine concentration is the nephrologist's and the Food and Drug Administration (FDA) advisory panel's favorite indicator of kidney function, treatment of ADPKD aimed at slowing disease progression cannot be tested in a formal, double-blind, placebo-controlled clinical trial until the serum creatinine level has begun to increase (i.e. glomerular filtration rate [GFR] is decreased). Unfortunately, a great deal of kidney damage has been done before the putative treatment can be tested, i.e., "the horse is out of the barn." Drugs like tolvaptan are aimed at targets causing the cysts to form and to grow; they will be most efficacious when started early in the course of ADPKD as confirmed in preclinical trials in animals with PKD. The potential impact of such drugs is lessened when administered late in the disease process when massive inflammation and scarring, which the "early drugs" can't alter, play major roles to promote the decline of glomerular filtration rate.

In the broad field of chronic, progressive kidney diseases, the FDA has established "hard endpoints:" death, dialysis or renal transplantation, for controlled clinical trials. In a successful trial, the research subjects given dummy medication (placebo) die, require dialysis or renal transplantation to a greater extent than those given the experimental drug. Neither the research subject nor the local care team knows who will receive the placebo or the candidate medication. Without the placebo group, we would never know for certain that the tested drug was doing any more than a sugar pill might achieve.

This procedure is the gold standard for determining if drugs do enough good to justify being put on the market. Unfortunately, in slowly progressive kidney disorders, demonstrating that a candidate drug extends life in comparison to a control group taking a placebo requires large numbers of volunteers willing to remain in the study for many years. The studies become frightfully expensive.

Prior to starting the Phase III trial, the treatment protocol had to be formally discussed with the FDA. Frank Czerwiec, M.D., Ph.D., Senior Director for Otsuka's Global Clinical Development group corporation, briefed the consultants on what to expect. I had never attended one of these meetings and was struck by the formal ambience from the moment I walked into the FDA building in Silver Spring, Maryland.

Everyone knew, coming into this meeting, that a prohibitively expensive, decades-long trial would be required if the FDA insisted that tolvaptan reduce the incidence of death, dialysis or renal transplantation in comparison to placebo. We hoped that sequential measurements of kidney volume and the hard outcome data in experimental animals would carry the day.

After passing though the security gate, we were ushered into a small room and asked to wait until summoned. Everyone spoke in hushed tones, as though they were afraid someone might be watching and listening through secret microphones or video. I remember thinking to myself that these Otsuka people must be reading too many spy novels. After an indeterminate wait, we were led into a dimly-lit meeting room and squeezed into a narrow space on one side of a long table opposite the FDA staff members on the other side, who had considerably more room to slouch or scoot their chairs about. The meeting started with perfunctory introductions by everyone in the room followed by the presentation of scientific evidence that had been gathered over the previous 20 years implicating vasopressin and cyclic AMP as major causes of disease progression in PKD. Because the disease caused the kidneys to progressively enlarge and tolvaptan slowed kidney growth and preserved renal function in several animal models of PKD, we thought that the efficacy of tolvaptan could be established in a controlled clinical trial if it lessened the rate that polycystic kidneys enlarged. Speakers explaining how tolvaptan would reduce disease progression gave it their best shot.

But when the Otsuka Corp. rested its case and the leader of the FDA panel rose to speak, we learned quickly that we had been shot down in a crashing heap before we had even lifted off. The evidence had not convinced the panel that Total Kidney Volume (TKV) was a "hard endpoint." In other words, the massive size some of the kidneys reached was not considered serious enough to warrant pharmacologic intervention. Nor was evidence that TKV could predict if or when a patient would develop kidney failure strong enough to authorize its use as a surrogate marker.

We had hit a brick wall! The room began to empty out to be replaced by the gloom of millions of disappointed patients with ADPKD all angry with me for failing them. At this point, Frank Czerwiec stepped forward and cautioned everyone to relax just a little bit and to not lose heart. He had detected some encouraging signs in the FDA's critique that tolvaptan might live to have another day in court.

Weeks later, I learned from Frank Czerwiec that the door had been left ajar to hear more about surrogate end-points, for example, an increase in the serum creatinine concentration. If a specified increase in the serum creatinine concentration was diminished by tolvaptan, that might be sufficient for approval. It would be necessary to recruit patients on the cusp of developing a declining GFR. The Phase II trials seemed to be proceeding well, so the OPCJ gave the "go ahead" for the Phase III, double-blind, placebo-controlled trial of tolvaptan with a goal of enrolling more than 1,400 patients. After further consultation with the FDA, progressive kidney enlargement would remain the primary endpoint (that would be largely ignored) and a composite secondary endpoint would include worsening kidney function, worsening hypertension, worsening albuminuria and severe kidney pain.

Neither the volunteers nor the medical staff looking after them would know if subjects got the real stuff or not. A few subjects would figure it out when they took the first pill and had to run to the bathroom in a couple of hours with a full urinary bladder. Those getting the drug developed a powerful thirst that forced them to drink upwards of 2 to 4 extra quarts of fluid each day. Recruitment of research volunteers took place around the globe. About one-quarter of the volunteers dropped out of the study, mostly because of the need to drink large amounts of water that often disturbed their sleep. The vast majority in the tolvaptan group took the drug for three years.

Encouraging developments during the Phase III trial buoyed expectations that tolvaptan would perform as hypothesized. Darren Wallace's lab published results showing that tolvaptan blocked vasopressin-dependent proliferation and net fluid secretion by cells removed from human cysts and grown in culture, strong evidence that these cells responded to the hormone and the inhibitor as postulated in the human trials.

In 2011, the Phase II "open-label" study of tolvaptan was completed and the results compared to patients in the long-term natural history study called CRISP. In a three-year period, tolvaptan slowed the rate of kidney enlargement by 71 percent and reduced the fall in glomerular filtration rate by 66 percent. Because the number of subjects was relatively small and a control group was not studied contemporaneously, the final results, though encouraging, could not be considered definitive. Any cheering and shouting would have to wait until the Phase III trial was completed.

CHAPTER 32

Promises kept

I made slow but steady progress to increase mobility and security afoot. My overarching goal for the rest of my life is to not fall, for I cannot rise from a prostrate position without assistance. We tend to underappreciate how important arms are in executing the innumerable tasks ordinary humans perform in the course of a day. "Need is the mother of invention" is an oft-recited quote; I have discovered a multitude of needs and quite a few inventions to compensate for the loss of arm function. Still, I need assistance with disrobing, showering and shaving in the mornings and with getting ready for the reclining chair at night. Workers' compensation takes care of the morning exercises and nurse Carol does the chores at night. The first Sunday I was able to attend a church service, while still decorated with my halo, I spoke to the congregation, thanking them for their prayers and other support. I also introduced a new concept to the Methodist Church by declaring sainthood for Carol. There was no dissent from the congregation.

The long recuperation gave me more time to think about urine, and more time to think specifically about the complex process of cyst formation in ADPKD. Larry Cook, Ph.D. helped me use data from the CRISP study to determine that renal cysts that develop in babies before they are born grow at extraordinarily rapid rates until the child is delivered. The growth rate of these early cysts declines after birth. We also determined that renal cysts are like icebergs; we can only see about 1 to 2 percent of them in MRI scanners; most hide below the limit of resolution, which is about 1 mm in diameter. This and other information enabled us to construct a general theory of renal cyst development and growth that should be helpful in the care of patients.

Since my latest shaping experience in the library, I have spent approximately six hours of each day, including Saturdays and Sundays, seated at a computer terminal, my index fingers pecking out text, making charts or exploring the world's scientific literature through PubMed and Google. I owe whatever sanity I have left to computers and the Internet, as the loss of physical mobility and dexterity has made it impossible to practice medicine or work in the laboratory.

In the spring of 2012, Frank Czerwiec and Holly Krasa, M.S., his collaborator in Rockville, Maryland, wanted to make a hasty visit to the Kidney Institute to meet with me regarding the recently completed Phase III trial of tolvaptan in patients with ADPKD. This was the ultimate "final test" of the hypothesis I had hatched a quarter of a century earlier and which was soon to be exposed as a proof of concept or a multimillion dollar dud. Czerwiec would not disclose beforehand the exact purpose of the visit, and he seemed unusually tense on the phone when we discussed the logistics of finding me in the cavernous Kansas University Medical Center. As a consultant, I was held to a confidentiality agreement not to discuss anything about the trial; my friend, Vicente Torres, the principal investigator of the Phase III study, had to operate by the same code of ethics, so I had nowhere to go to find out what the data had revealed.

I began to worry that a problem had turned up in the final data analysis or that patients had suffered some calamity because they took tolvaptan. I had several sleepless nights before Czerwiec and Krasa arrived on campus, and we met in my office with the door closed. Dr. Czerwiec explained that they had completed the data analysis and were interested in my impressions. They wanted to be with me when I saw the data firsthand so that questions could be addressed immediately. They were especially interested in my opinion about the final conclusions.

Over the next hour, I examined detailed data displays and graphs that were used to portray the major effects of the drug spanning a three-year course in more than 1,400 volunteers with ADPKD. As the data unfolded, it became unmistakably clear that this study had reached the goal I had been pursuing 24/7 since the intrusive memory of Ronnie Wilkerson's bleeding kidneys led me into PKD research. The struggle to gain a therapeutic foothold on PKD while battling peers in renal research who favored other agendas, working to establish and to insure the credibility of the PKDF, the innumerable "rubber chicken dinners" eaten away from my family while advocating for PKD research on the lecture circuit, the weighty sense of responsibility to Ronnie and the thousands of individuals with PKD whose hopes for treatment I helped to raise and to those who had pledged their financial treasure in support of this crusade — suddenly, this all stormed down on me as the last bits of data were revealed. I fought back tears as the realization of a successful outcome swept over me, and I slapped my better hand on the table and shouted out words I can't recall. Frank told me sometime later that he and Holly expected no less of an emotional response. In fact, that is why they came to Kansas City rather than discussing the triumph on the telephone. They wanted to witness my response.

The results were unambiguous and spectacularly positive. Tolvaptan had slowed the rate of increase in kidney size by nearly 50 percent and the rate of decline in glomerular filtration by 31 percent, strong evidence proving that ADPKD can be effectively treated by drugs targeting specific components of the cyst growth process — a proof of principle. For this "Brother of the Cysterhood," the manuscript written by Vicente Torres, M.D., Cysterhood brother of the highest order, and published in the prestigious "New England Journal of Medicine in December 2012," represented the end of the beginning.

❖

EPILOGUE

Thanks to the intellectual and physical contributions of exceptionally committed basic and physician scientists around the world, we have
reached this important milestone, and I have made a down payment on
promises to two of my closest childhood friends: to Ronnie Wilkerson I
had vowed to do something to mitigate the untimely loss of his life to
polycystic kidney disease; to Donnie Richard, whose life ended prematurely in an iron lung, I had sworn to live for both of us. Carol and our
children can take some ownership in the successful outcome of this decades-long quest that often left them with a pre-occupied husband and
father. My strongest regret is that I robbed my family of precious moments
together at important times in their lives. Thankfully, barring any more
shaping experiences, I still have a little time left to make amends to those
I love so deeply, although, in the reverie of a late night or early morning,
would it be considered a sin to think about urine — just a little bit?

There once was a man, Jared Grantham,
Whose life would sing loudly this anthem:
"About the urine — I think"
"But it's the water you drink"
"That holds cures for all cyst expansion."

James P. Calvet, Ph.D.